Kidney Transplantation

Remedica State of the Art series
ISSN 1472-4626

Also available
The Handbook of Diabetes Mellitus and Cardiovascular Disease
The Inflammatory Bowel Disease Yearbook
Management of Atherosclerotic Carotid Disease
Management of Peripheral Arterial Disease
Multiple Myeloma
Rheumatoid Arthritis
Viral Co-infections in HIV: Impact and Management

Published by the Remedica Group
Remedica Publishing Ltd, 32–38 Osnaburgh Street, London, NW1 3ND, UK
Remedica Inc, Tri State International Center, Building 25, Suite 150,
Lincolnshire, IL 60069, USA

Email: books@remedica.com
www.remedica.com

Publisher: Andrew Ward
In-house editor: Cath Harris

ISBN 1 901346 49 8
British Library Cataloguing-in-Publication Data
A catalogue record for this book is available from the British Library

Kidney Transplantation

Donald E Hricik, Editor

Professor, CWRU
Residency Program Director, UHHS
University Hospitals of Cleveland
11100 Euclid Avenue
Room 8124 Lakeside Building
Cleveland, OH 44106
USA

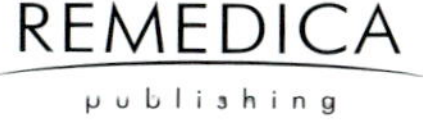

LONDON • CHICAGO

Contributors

Kenneth A Bodziak, MD
Case Western Reserve University, 11100 Euclid Avenue, Cleveland, OH 44106, USA

Peter S Heeger, MD
The Department of Immunology and the Urologic Institute, The Cleveland Clinic Foundation, 9500 Euclid Avenue, NB30, Cleveland, OH 44195, USA

J Harold Helderman, MD
Nephrology Division, Vanderbilt University, 2201 West End Avenue, Nashville, TN 37235, USA

Donald E Hricik, MD
Case Western Reserve University, 11100 Euclid Avenue, Room 8124 Lakeside Building, Cleveland, OH 44106, USA

Anthony Langone, MD
Nephrology Division, S-3223 MCN, Vanderbilt University Medical Center, Nashville, TN 37232, USA

Mariana Markell, MD
Division of Renal Diseases, SUNY Downstate Medical Center, Box 52, 450 Clarkson Avenue, Brooklyn, NY 11203, USA

John D Pirsch, MD
Division of Organ Transplantation University of Wisconsin Medical School, H4/772 Clinical Science Center, 600 Highland Avenue, Madison, WI 53792, USA

Moro O Salifu, MD
Department of Internal Medicine, Division of Nephrology, SUNY Downstate Medical Center, Brooklyn, NY 11203, USA

James Schulak, MD
Chairman, Department of Surgery, Case Western Reserve University, University Hospitals of Cleveland, Department of Surgery, 11100 Euclid Avenue, Cleveland, OH 44106, USA

John F Valente, MD
Renal Transplant Program, Case Western Reserve University, University Hospitals of Cleveland, Department of Surgery, 11100 Euclid Avenue, Cleveland, OH 44106, USA

Preface

Short-term outcomes in kidney transplantation have dramatically improved in recent history. This reflects a better understanding of the immune mechanisms that lead to allograft rejection, and the development of potent new regimens of immunosuppressive drugs that effectively prevent and treat rejection. Concurrent surgical innovations have included techniques for harvesting multiple organs, laparoscopic organ removal, and strategies for the surgical management of marginal donors and recipients who would have been rejected in an earlier era.

The long-term survival of renal allografts has been increasingly influenced by nonimmune factors, and death with a functioning graft has emerged as the most common cause of late allograft failure. Thus, attention has turned to strategies that optimize long-term allograft survival by minimizing the toxicities of immunosuppressants. These contribute to infection, malignancy, chronic renal dysfunction, and cardiovascular disease – the major causes of posttransplant mortality.

With increasing rates of success, the number of kidney transplant recipients continues to expand worldwide. Increasingly, medical personnel from a variety of subspecialties will be exposed to these patients and participate in their care. This book provides a concise review of the current status of kidney transplantation, and will help to update physicians, trainees, nurses, and other professionals who either care for patients with kidney disease or who are interested in organ transplantation.

Chapter 1 summarizes recent trends in kidney transplant outcomes, and also delineates the disturbing and growing disparity between the number of potential kidney transplant recipients and the number of available organs.

In Chapter 2, current understanding of the immunology of acute and chronic allograft rejection is reviewed as the basis for modern immunosuppression protocols. During the past decade, a plethora of new immunosuppressive drugs has become available for the prevention and treatment of acute renal allograft rejection. The advantages and disadvantages of the newer drugs and drug combinations are summarized in Chapter 3.

In the past decade, selection criteria for potential kidney transplant recipients have been expanded and revised. With increasing waiting times for cadaveric allografts, re-evaluation of patients who are on the waiting list for prolonged periods of time has become imperative. Current criteria for selection of kidney transplant recipients, re-evaluation of wait-listed patients, and the evaluation of living donors are reviewed in Chapter 4.

Chapter 5 provides an update on surgical techniques for harvesting kidneys from both cadaveric and living donors, and also reviews the management of common surgical complications of kidney transplantation.

Finally, Chapter 6 reviews the pathophysiology and management of the most common long-term complications of kidney transplantation, including cardiovascular disease, infection, bone disease, and malignancy.

It is the hope of the authors that this book will stimulate interest in the field of kidney transplantation, and ultimately lead to better care of kidney transplant recipients.

Donald Hricik
Case Western Reserve University

Contents

Chapter 1: Recent trends in kidney transplantation 1
Kenneth A Bodziak & Donald E Hricik

Chapter 2: Transplantation immunology 13
Peter S Heeger

Chapter 3: Immunosuppressive drug therapy 39
Anthony J Langone & J Harold Helderman

Chapter 4: Evaluation of kidney transplant recipients and donors 55
Moro O Salifu & Mariana S Markell

Chapter 5: Surgical considerations in kidney transplantation 79
John F Valente & James A Schulak

Chapter 6: Long-term complications of kidney transplantion 97
John D Pirsch

Abbreviations 117

Index 119

1

Recent trends in kidney transplantation

Kenneth A Bodziak & Donald E Hricik

Introduction

Kidney transplantation has emerged as the renal replacement therapy of choice for patients with end-stage renal disease (ESRD) who lack comorbidities that preclude elective surgery or the rigors of chronic immunosuppression. An analysis of the US Renal Data System (USRDS) database computed "projected years of life" for primary cadaveric kidney transplant recipients, and compared them with age-matched patients maintained on dialysis while waiting for a kidney transplant [1]. This analysis indicated that kidney transplantation offers a survival advantage over treatment with dialysis for all age groups (see **Table 1**). The advantage is particularly striking in young patients and in those with diabetes mellitus. Unfortunately, the growing disparity between the number of patients waiting for organs and the number of organs available means that kidney transplantation can be offered to an increasingly small proportion of the ESRD population.

This introductory chapter reviews the current outcomes of kidney transplantation, problems created by the organ-donor shortage, and recent trends in immunosuppression.

Trends in kidney transplant volume and donor source

During the past decade, the number of kidney transplants performed annually in the US has remained relatively fixed at approximately 13,000 per year. As shown in **Figure 1**, the small

Age (years), diabetes status	Projected years of life	
	Wait-listed patients	Transplanted patients
20–39, no diabetes	20	31
20–39, diabetes	8	25
40–59, no diabetes	12	19
40–59, diabetes	8	22
60–74, no diabetes	7	12
60–74, diabetes	5	8

Table 1. Comparison of life expectancies of wait-listed dialysis patients versus primary transplant recipients. Reproduced with permission from the Massachusetts Medical Society (*N Engl J Med* 1999;341:1725–30).

growth in the annual number of kidney transplants performed between 1990 and 2000 has resulted almost entirely from an increase in the number of transplants performed using living donors. The number of transplants performed using cadaver donors has remained fixed at approximately 8,000 per year.

During the same period of time, liberalization of the criteria for acceptance to dialysis programs has resulted in continuous growth in the ESRD patient population. The expected consequences of the imbalance between supply and demand are as follows: an exponential increase in the number of patients waiting for a transplant (see **Figure 1**); an increase in waiting times; and an increase in the number of patients who die while waiting for a transplant. Median waiting times approximately tripled between 1988 and 1998 [2]; mortality rates for patients on the US waiting list increased from 3.7% in 1988 to 4.7% in 2000 [3]; and in 1999 alone, 3,088 patients with ESRD died in the US while waiting for a kidney transplant [3].

Living donors

The recent increase in the use of living donors has been motivated, in part, by the long waiting times for cadaver organs, and is ethically justified by steadily improving outcomes for kidney

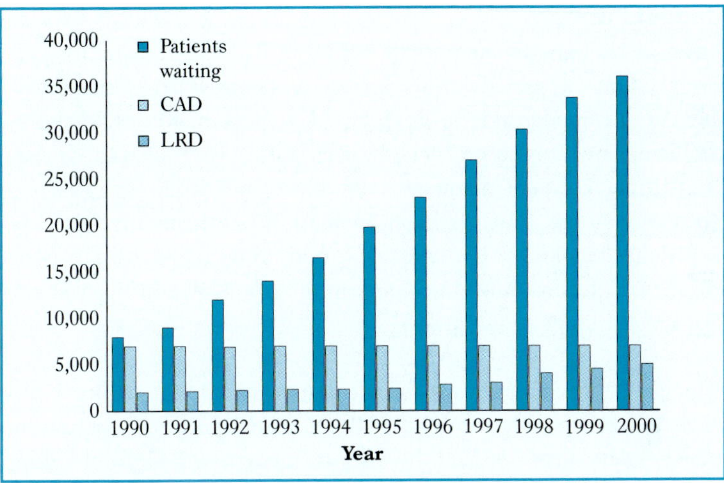

Figure 1. Number of kidney transplants performed and patients waiting for cadaveric transplants between 1990 and 2000. CAD: cadaveric donor transplants; LRD: living-related donor transplants.

transplant recipients. While living relatives (ie, members of the nuclear family) are still the most common source of living donors, the number of transplants performed with living "unrelated" donors (eg, spouses or friends) has dramatically increased during the past decade.

Allografts from living unrelated donors exhibit survival rates that exceed those from cadaver donors with equivalent degrees of human leukocyte antigen (HLA) matching, and approach those of zero-mismatched cadaveric donors [4,5]. This suggests that the benefit of eliminating cold ischemia in the case of living donor transplantation outweighs the immunologic disadvantages of HLA mismatching, and has fueled efforts to expand the living-donor pool by identifying both emotionally related and emotionally unrelated living donors [6]. Laparoscopic techniques for performing donor nephrectomies (see Chapter 5) have shortened the period of postoperative rehabilitation for living kidney donors [7], and provide additional motivation for promoting living donor kidney transplantation.

Cadaver donors

Attempts to expand the pool of kidneys from cadaver donors have centered on the use of donors previously deemed to be "marginal" due to advanced age, a history of hypertension or diabetes mellitus, prolonged cold-ischemia time, or elevated serum creatinine concentration at the time of organ harvesting. Transplantation of two kidneys instead of one from such donors, in order to maximize the mass of functioning nephrons, has been employed in an effort to use organs that would have been discarded in a previous era [8].

A logical concern regarding the use of marginal donors is that long-term outcomes may be negatively affected. However, analysis of USRDS data indicates that the long-term survival benefit of kidney transplantation persists in recipients of kidneys from marginal donors [9]. Results from this analysis undoubtedly contributed to a recent decision by the United Network for Organ Sharing to create a separate kidney transplant waiting list for recipients willing to accept organs based on "expanded donor criteria".

Current allograft and patient outcomes

Recent trends in kidney transplantation have led to a dramatic improvement in short-term outcomes, including a marked decline in the incidence of early acute rejection episodes, and 1-year graft survival rates that exceed 90% in many centers.

These improvements reflect a better understanding of the immune mechanisms that lead to rejection of an allograft, and the development of immunosuppressants that effectively prevent and treat rejection. The availability of effective prophylaxis against cytomegalovirus and other pathogens undoubtedly has contributed to lower rates of acute rejection by allowing relatively potent immunosuppression during the first few months after transplantation without an excessive risk of infectious complications.

Donor source	Projected graft half-life (years)			
	Before death censoring			
	1988	1991	1993	1995
Living	12.7	14.8	16.7	21.6
Cadaveric	7.9	9.7	10.3	13.8
	After death censoring			
Living	16.9	21.5	22.9	35.9
Cadaveric	11.0	14.5	15.1	19.5

Table 2. Projected half-life of renal transplants, 1988–1995. Reproduced with permission from the Massachusetts Medical Society (*N Engl J Med* 2000;342:605–12).

Early acute rejection

In the late 1980s, around 60% of kidney transplant recipients experienced at least one episode of acute allograft rejection during the first year following transplantation. By 2001, the incidence of early acute rejection had decreased to below 20% in many centers, presumably reflecting the potency of new immunosuppressant drugs and drug combinations. As a consequence of improvements in the short-term outcomes of renal allografts, benchmarks for success in kidney transplantation have shifted from conventional measures, such as 1-year graft survival or the incidence of early acute rejection, to measures such as allograft half-life or survival rates beyond 5 years.

Because acute rejection is a strong independent correlate of chronic allograft dysfunction and graft loss [10,11], the decline in the frequency of acute rejection is expected to extend the lives of renal allografts. Indeed, the half-lives of transplanted kidneys gradually increased among patients who were transplanted between 1988 and 1995: the projected half-life of a living-donor transplanted kidney increased from 12.7 years to 21.6 years during this time period, while the half-life of a cadaver-donor kidney increased from 7.9 years to 13.8 years (see **Table 2**) [12]. After censoring for death with a functioning graft, in 1995, the projected half-lives were 35.9 years for living-donor kidneys and 19.5 years for cadaver-donor kidneys.

In this analysis, an episode of acute rejection within the first year after transplantation was found to have a detrimental effect on long-term graft survival. Over the 7-year study period, the average yearly reduction in the relative risk of graft failure was 6.3% for patients who never had an episode of acute rejection, and 0.4% for those who did [12].

A further analysis of USRDS data suggested that, during the late 1990s, an early acute rejection episode had an even greater negative impact on long-term graft survival than it did in the late 1980s [13]. Compared with a reference group of patients who were transplanted in 1988–1989 with no rejection, having an acute rejection episode in 1988–1989, 1992–1993, and 1996–1997 conferred, respectively, a 1.7-fold, 3.4-fold, and 5.2-fold relative risk for the subsequent development of graft failure [13]. Thus, despite declining incidence, acute rejection remains a problem and eradication of early rejection episodes remains a laudable goal.

Chronic allograft nephropathy

Acute rejection is among several predictors of chronic rejection, which is one of the leading causes of late allograft failure. In fact, the term "chronic rejection" has been replaced with "chronic allograft nephropathy" (CAN), to emphasize that both immune and nonimmune mechanisms play a pathophysiologic role in this process. Histologically, CAN is characterized by interstitial fibrosis, glomerulosclerosis, and vascular neointimal hyperplasia and fibrosis. Clinical correlates of this lesion include progressive deterioration of renal function, worsening hypertension, and proteinuria.

Nonimmune factors that may contribute to CAN and its underlying pathology include systemic hypertension, hyperlipidemia, nephrotoxicity mediated by calcineurin inhibitors (ie, cyclosporine or tacrolimus), viral infections, and ischemia-reperfusion injury. CAN currently accounts for approximately 30% of late renal allograft failures, and is now the fourth most common cause of ESRD

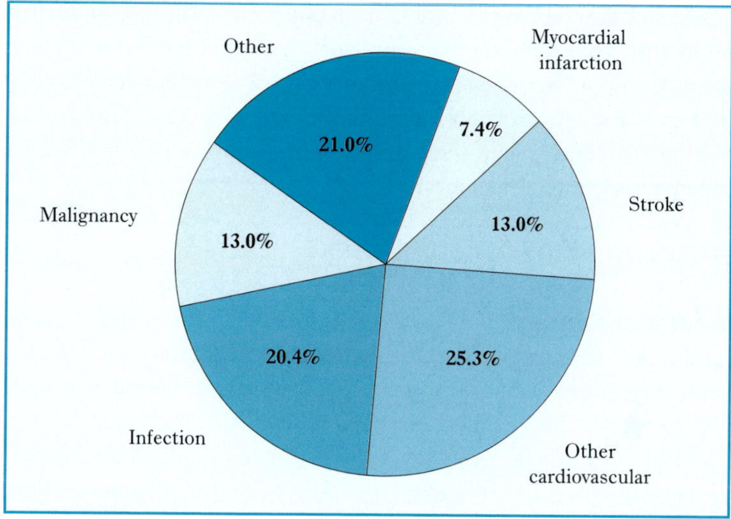

Figure 2. Causes of death in renal transplant recipients with functioning allografts (1995–1997). Adapted from the US Renal Data System 1999 Annual Data Report.

(after diabetes mellitus, hypertension, and glomerulonephritis) among patients on the cadaveric transplant waiting list.

Death from cardiovascular disease

Death with a functioning allograft is the most common cause of late allograft failure in many transplant centers [14]. In the past 15 years, cardiovascular disease (including myocardial infarction, stroke, and complications of peripheral vascular disease) has emerged as the leading cause of mortality in kidney transplant recipients (see **Figure 2**). However, it is important to note that the incidence of death from cardiovascular disease after kidney transplantation is much lower than that in dialysis patients. In one registry analysis, annual mortality from cardiovascular disease was 9.1% in hemodialysis patients, 0.54% in transplant recipients, and 0.28% in the general population [15].

A very high prevalence of posttransplant hypertension, hyperlipidemia, and diabetes mellitus undoubtedly contributes to cardiovascular morbidity and mortality in kidney transplant recipients (see Chapter 6). Ironically, many of the most widely used immunosuppressants enhance these cardiovascular risk factors, and are therefore likely to play an important pathophysiologic role in the development of cardiovascular disease following kidney transplantation.

Trends in immunosuppression

Induction therapy

"Induction therapy" using antilymphocyte antibodies to prevent acute rejection during the early posttransplant period remains controversial. Both polyclonal and monoclonal antibodies are available for induction therapy. In virtually all clinical trials, use of such antibodies has reduced the risk of acute rejection when compared with placebo. However, the benefits of induction antibodies must be weighed against the considerable cost of these agents, and concern that they may increase the risk of over-immunosuppression. Some transplant centers now reserve induction therapy for patients deemed to be at high risk for acute rejection, eg, African Americans, nonprimary transplant recipients, patients with high titers of anti-HLA antibodies, and recipients of simultaneous pancreas–kidney transplants.

Immunosuppressive drugs

In the 1990s, the development of several new immunosuppressive drugs made it possible to design maintenance immunosuppression regimens based on an individual patient's comorbid conditions or estimated immunologic risk of rejection. With improvements in short-term outcomes, attention has increasingly turned to strategies that optimize long-term allograft survival by minimizing the side effects of immunosuppressants.

The aim is to prolong patient survival by reducing the risks of infection, malignancy, chronic renal dysfunction, and cardiovascular disease. Thus, while many transplant centers begin maintenance immunosuppression with a combination of two or three drugs (see Chapter 3), enthusiasm is increasing for protocols that intentionally reduce immunosuppression over time, or that convert patients to new drugs in order to eliminate the toxicities of a prior regimen.

Recent efforts have focused on protocols that either avoid, withdraw, or minimize exposure to calcineurin inhibitors in an attempt to eliminate the chronic nephrotoxicity and cardiovascular toxicities associated with these agents [16–18]. There has also been renewed enthusiasm for protocols in which corticosteroids are either avoided or withdrawn [19]. The benefits of these minimization strategies must be weighed against the risks of precipitating acute or chronic allograft rejection.

Future directions

Although modern immunosuppression has been associated with improved outcomes in kidney transplant recipients, currently employed immunosuppressive drugs remain nonspecific, posing a constant risk of over-immunosuppression, with neoplasia and infection as the most feared consequences.

Immunosuppression

To a large extent, dosing of immunosuppressive drugs is empiric. For some agents, therapeutic drug monitoring can guide dosing; however, measurement of drug levels in the blood does not provide an accurate assessment of the patient's overall state of immunosuppression. Currently, allograft rejection is recognized clinically by a rising serum creatinine concentration, and confirmed histologically by renal biopsy.

The recognition that acute rejection can occur histologically without clinical manifestations raises the concern that some patients may be chronically under-immunosuppressed, and has stimulated interest in the use of serial "surveillance" biopsies to rule-out subclinical rejection [20]. Obviously, a noninvasive assay that could monitor a patient's level of immunosuppression and/or serve as a surrogate for acute rejection would enhance the management of kidney transplant recipients. Although a number of tests are being investigated (eg, blood or urine cytokine profiles, mixed lymphocyte reactions, urine spectroscopy, microarrays) [21], none has yet proven sufficiently sensitive or specific to serve as a clinical standard of practice.

Immunologic tolerance

Immunologic tolerance – a state in which a transplant recipient requires no immunosuppression, fails to reject a donor's organ, but remains immunologically responsive to third parties (such as pathogens) – has been called the "Holy Grail" of transplantation, and is the focus of a great deal of basic and clinical research.

While readily achieved in small animal models, true tolerance has been difficult to reach in humans. Complete ablation of the bone marrow and bone marrow transplantation can result in true tolerance to a subsequent organ transplanted from the same donor [22], but the inherent dangers of marrow eradication and transplantation preclude widespread clinical applicability.

Basic research into immunologic tolerance has focused on the recognition of costimulatory T-cell signals, which, when blocked, lead to T-cell apoptosis or anergy (see Chapter 2). Ongoing clinical research has emphasized the use of nonablative, lymphocyte-depleting regimens (with or without supplemental donor-derived bone marrow transplantation), which may facilitate a state of immunologic hyporesponsiveness, if not true tolerance.

Inducing a state of true tolerance would theoretically remove the need for toxic immunosuppressants, and also eliminate immunologic rejection as a cause of graft loss. However, even this would not correct the imbalance between organ supply and demand. Xenotransplantation (transplantation across species) could alleviate the problem and is a focus of intense research. Although some of the immunologic hurdles of xeno-transplantation have been overcome through genetic engineering of animals, severe rejection remains a limiting factor [23]. Concerns regarding the transmission of infectious diseases and whether or not a xenotransplant can sustain normal physiology for long periods of time are additional reasons why xenotransplantation has not yet become a clinical reality.

Conclusion

The field of renal transplantation has witnessed a marked improvement in both short- and long-term outcomes. However, as the number of patients with ESRD increases, the demand for organs continues to rise, and growth in living-donor transplantation has not sufficiently offset the need. Achieving immunologic tolerance and performing successful xenotransplantation currently form the basis of intense research.

References

1. Wolfe RA, Ashby VB, Milford EL et al. Comparison of mortality in all patients on dialysis, patients on dialysis awaiting transplantation, and recipients of a first cadaveric transplant. *N Engl J Med* 1999;341:1725–30.
2. Harper AM, Edwards EB, Ellison MD. The OPTN waiting list. In: Cecka JM, Terasaki PI, editors. *Clinical Transplants*. Los Angeles: UCLA Tissue Typing Laboratory, 2001:73–85.
3. United Network for Organ Sharing (UNOS). Available from URL: http://www.UNOS.org.
4. Terasaki PI, Cecka JM, Gjertson DW et al. High survival rates of kidney transplants from spousal and living unrelated donors. *N Engl J Med* 1995;333:333–6.
5. Gjertson DW, Cecka JM. Living unrelated donor kidney transplantation. *Kidney Int* 2000;58:491–9.
6. Matas AJ, Garvey CA, Jacobs CL et al. Nondirected donation of kidneys from living donors. *N Engl J Med* 2000;343:433–6.
7. Schweitzer EJ, Wilson J, Jacobs J et al. Increased rates of donation with laparoscopic donor nephrectomy. *Ann Surg* 2000;232:392–400.
8. Lu AD, Carter JT, Weinstein RJ et al. Outcome in recipients of dual kidney transplants: an analysis of the dual registry patients. *Transplantation* 2000;69:281–5.
9. Ojo AO, Hanson JA, Meier-Kriesche H et al. Survival in recipients of marginal cadaveric donor kidneys compared with other recipients and wait-listed transplant candidates. *J Am Soc Nephrol* 2001;12:589–97.
10. Cosio FG, Pelletier RP, Falkenhain ME et al. Impact of acute rejection and early allograft function on renal allograft survival. *Transplantation* 1997;63:1611–5.
11. Matas AJ, Humar A, Gillingham KJ et al. Five preventable causes of kidney graft loss in the 1990s: a single center analysis. *Kidney Int* 2002;62:704–14.
12. Hariharan S, Johnson CP, Bresnahan BA et al. Improved graft survival after renal transplantation in the United States, 1988 to 1996. *N Engl J Med* 2000;342:605–12.

13. Meier-Kriesche HU, Ojo AO, Hanson JA et al. Increased impact of acute rejection on chronic allograft failure in the recent era. *Transplantation* 2000;70:1098–100.
14. Kasiske BL, Chakkera HA, Roel J. Explained and unexplained ischemic heart disease risk after kidney transplantation. *J Am Soc Nephrol* 2000;11:1735–43.
15. Foley RN, Parfrey PS, Sarnak MJ. Epidemiology of cardiovascular disease in chronic renal disease. *J Am Soc Nephrol* 1998;9(12 Suppl.):S16–S23.
16. Weir MR, Ward MT, Blahut SA et al. Long-term impact of discontinued or reduced calcineurin inhibitors in patients with chronic allograft nephropathy. *Kidney Int* 2001;59:1567–73.
17. Morales JM, Wramner L, Kreis H et al. Sirolimus does not exhibit nephrotoxicity compared to cyclosporine in renal transplant recipients. *Am J Transplant* 2002;2:436–42.
18. Johnson RW, Kreis H, Oberbauer R et al. Sirolimus allows early cyclosporine withdrawal in renal transplantation resulting in improved renal function and lower blood pressure. *Transplantation* 2001;72:777–86.
19. Hricik DE. Steroid-free immunosuppression in kidney transplantation: an editorial review. *Am J Transplant* 2002;2:19–24.
20. Rush D, Somorjai R, Deslauriers R et al. Subclinical rejection – a potential surrogate marker for chronic rejection – may be diagnosed by protocol biopsy or urine spectroscopy. *Ann Transplant* 2000;5:44–9.
21. Hricik DE, Heeger PS. Minimization of immunosuppression in kidney transplantation: the need for immune monitoring. *Transplantation* 2001;72(8 Suppl.):S32–S35.
22. Dey B, Sykes M, Spitzer TR. Outcomes of recipients of both bone marrow and solid organ transplants. A review. *Medicine (Baltimore)* 1998;77:355–69.
23. Cascalho M, Platt JL. The immunological barrier to xenotransplantation. *Immunity* 2001;14:437–46.

2

Transplantation immunology

Peter S Heeger

Introduction

Transplantation has become the treatment of choice for end-stage kidney, liver, heart, and lung disease, and is being explored as a therapy for the failure of a variety of other organs. The major hurdle to successful transplantation is immune-mediated rejection, a process that has been partially prevented by the use of potent immunosuppressive medications [1,2]. The extraordinary strength of the immune response to a transplanted organ has fascinated immunologists and clinicians for decades [3], and is only now beginning to be understood in detail.

This chapter summarizes what is currently understood of this immune response in order to provide a foundation upon which to base rational clinical decisions aimed at prolonging graft survival. It is important to understand the immunologic basis of transplant rejection in order to comprehend the role of the tissue-typing laboratory in managing potential transplant recipients, to understand the mechanisms of immunosuppression, and to be able to detect and diagnose clinical transplantation rejection. Moreover, a sound immunologic foundation will permit the astute clinician to make the best use of new immune-based manipulations aimed at prolonging graft survival, and to evaluate novel surrogate markers for predicting both short-term and long-term outcomes.

Overview

Immune responses can be divided into humoral (ie, B cells and antibodies) and cellular (ie, T cells) components, both of which are involved in mediating transplant rejection. Following the transplant procedure, recipient T and B cells recognize donor antigens [1–6], usually within the secondary lymphoid organs (the draining lymph nodes or the spleen). The molecular and cellular basis of allorecognition by T cells, B cells, and antibodies is discussed in detail below.

Placement of an isograft – that is, an organ that is immunologically identical between donor and recipient (such as from one identical twin to another) – does not result in an immune response. Most grafts are transplanted from one member of a species to a nonidentical member of that same species (eg, from one human to another); these are termed "allografts". Under these circumstances, the two individuals differ at major histocompatibility complex (MHC) loci (known as human leukocyte antigen [HLA] loci in humans), and the transplant results in a potent antidonor alloimmune response.

If the T or B cell specifically recognizes an alloantigen under appropriate conditions, full activation and differentiation ensues (see **Figure 1**) [7]. Lymphocyte (T or B cell) activation results in production and secretion of new proteins (including cytokines and antibodies), alterations in the expression of cell surface molecules that direct cell migration, and proliferation.

Activated T cells are able to circulate through the peripheral organs, including the transplant itself. Chemoattractant proteins (chemokines) help to attract and accumulate donor antigen-specific T cells within the graft. Then, upon re-encounter with specific antigens in the graft itself, donor-reactive T cells make use of a wide variety of effector mechanisms that can result in acute graft destruction and/or chronic scarring and fibrosis.

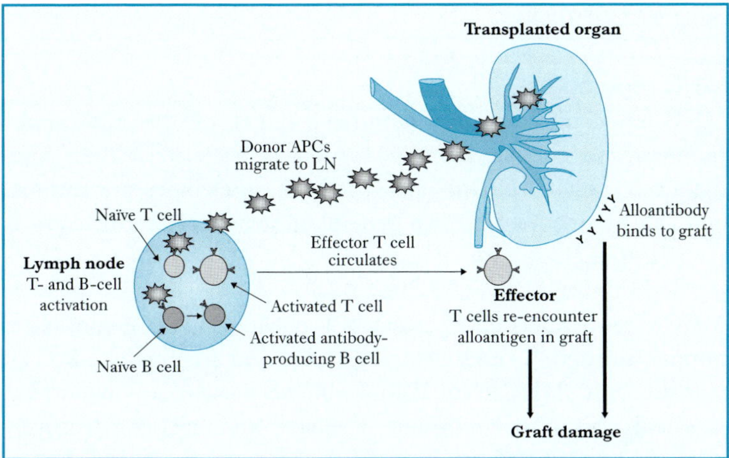

Figure 1. An overview of transplantation immunity. Following transplantation, donor-derived antigen-presenting cells (APCs) migrate to the recipient's lymph nodes (LN) or spleen and prime recipient T and B cells. Activated T cells differentiate into effector cells, alter cell surface molecule expression, and migrate to the peripheral tissues, including the donor organ. Activated B cells produce alloantibodies that can bind directly to major histocompatibility complex molecules expressed on the donor tissue. Local effector mechanisms ultimately result in destruction of the graft.

Similarly, circulating antibodies specific for donor HLA molecules (alloantibodies) produced by alloreactive B cells can interact with ligands expressed by cells in the graft, and trigger a variety of cellular and molecular effector mechanisms. If left untreated, these T-cell- and B-cell-mediated processes will together result in organ destruction and failure (see **Figure 1**).

In the following sections, the various phases of the transplant-induced immune response (allorecognition, activation, migration, and effector functions) are discussed in detail.

Allorecognition

MHC molecules

MHC molecules are the dominant target of the alloreactive humoral and cellular immune responses because of their high degree of polymorphism [5,6,8,9]. MHC molecules are dimers, and can be divided into two general subtypes: class I or class II (see **Figure 2**).

MHC class I molecules consist of a polymorphic α chain and a nonpolymorphic β_2-microglobulin chain, and are expressed on all somatic cells. MHC class II molecules consist of a polymorphic α chain and a polymorphic β chain, and are constitutively expressed on a small number of antigen-presenting cells (APCs; eg, dendritic cells, B cells, macrophages). They can also be upregulated on many other cell types (eg, renal tubular cells) in the context of inflammation.

All MHC molecules contain a binding groove in which peptides are noncovalently bound. The peptides derive from either intracellular (generally expressed on MHC I) or extracellular (generally expressed on MHC II) proteins. MHC–peptide complexes are expressed on the cell surface where they present antigens to T cells.

MHC genes and gene products

There are several different genetic loci for each class of MHC molecule, and there are many polymorphisms at each locus. These polymorphisms predominantly fall within the peptide-binding grooves, such that different alleles bind to different repertoires of peptides. Thus, each species expresses a huge diversity of MHC molecules, allowing the species as a whole to respond to an enormous number of peptide antigens [5,6,9].

As noted above, in humans, the MHC complex is also called the HLA complex [9]. HLA class I A, B, and C loci are routinely studied by tissue-typing laboratories. HLA A2 and HLA A3 are

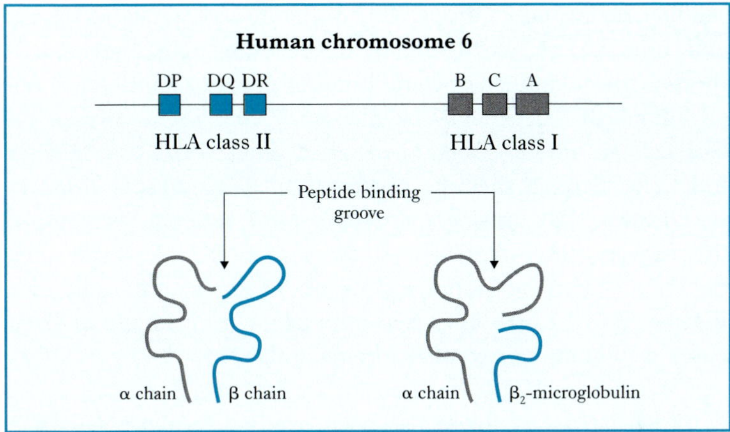

Figure 2. Major histocompatibility complex molecules are the primary targets of the alloimmune response. Human leukocyte antigen (HLA) molecules are encoded for on human chromosome 6. The class I loci (A, B, and C) encode polymorphic α chains that combine with β_2-microglobulin to produce an intact HLA class I molecule. The class II loci (DP, DQ, and DR) encode polymorphic α and β chains that combine to produce intact HLA class II molecules.

examples of two different HLA polymorphisms at the A locus, and differ by a number of amino acids (though the overall structures of the two molecules are quite similar). The predominant HLA class II loci are DP, DQ, and DR. DR1 and DR3 are representative of polymorphisms at the DR locus.

Humoral immunity: alloantibodies

Antibodies are produced by activated B cells, and are comprised of two covalently attached heavy chains and two light chains [5]. Antibody structure can be schematically envisioned as being Y-shaped. The base of the "Y" represents the constant, or Fc, region of the antibody (formed by two heavy chains). It is important for binding to complement, macrophages, and natural killer (NK) cells, thus mediating effector functions.

The two upper portions of the "Y", comprised of heavy and light chain regions, represent the highly polymorphic bivalent antigen-binding region (see **Figure 3A**). Antibodies generally recognize and bind to nonself (foreign) three-dimensional structures through these antigen-specific binding domains. Antibodies are evolutionarily "designed" to recognize foreign structures on extracellular invading organisms, and elicit secondary effector functions through their Fc receptors to destroy these invaders (see **Figure 3B**). Analogously, alloreactive antibodies recognize the foreign, three-dimensional structures of the polymorphic regions of HLA molecules expressed on donor graft cells (see **Figure 3C**). In principle, this interaction is no different from antibody binding to any other foreign antigen.

If the transplant recipient has been exposed to allogeneic HLA molecules through a blood transfusion, pregnancy, or previous transplant, then donor-reactive alloantibodies may be present prior to transplant [10–13]. This can predispose the patient to hyperacute rejection of the organ, and for this reason pretransplant antibody crossmatch studies are performed. High titers of donor-reactive alloantibodies are generally contraindicative to kidney transplantation from that donor (though this is not an absolute contraindication for heart or lung transplantation) [10–13]. Alloantibodies can additionally develop after transplantation, and may contribute to the development of acute and chronic rejection.

Allorecognition by T cells

T cells recognize MHC–peptide complexes through heterodimeric T-cell receptors (TCR) expressed on their cell surface. T cells can be divided into two broad subtypes based on the expression of one of two coreceptors: CD4 or CD8.

The CD4 and CD8 molecules help to stabilize the interaction between a TCR and its MHC–peptide ligand, and furthermore define whether the T cell can interact with peptides expressed in the context of MHC class I versus MHC class II molecules. CD4+ T cells recognize MHC II–peptide complexes [2,5,6], while CD8+ T cells recognize MHC I–peptide complexes.

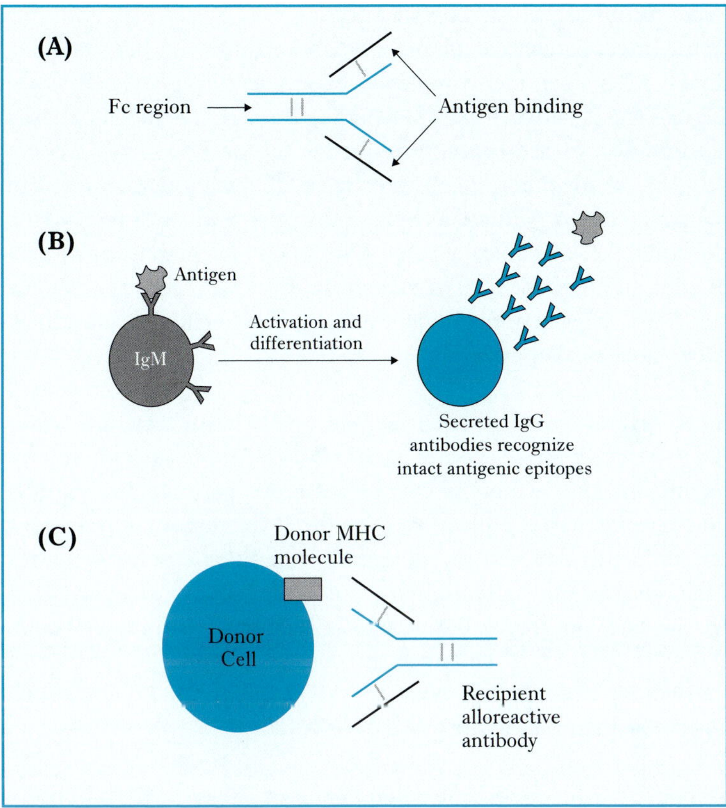

Figure 3. Antibody production in response to exogenous antigen. (**A**) Antibodies are comprised of highly polymorphic antigen-binding regions and an Fc region that mediates effector functions. (**B**) Intact antigens are recognized by immunoglobulin (Ig)M surface receptors expressed on B cells, resulting in differentiation of an antibody-secreting plasma cell. (**C**) An alloantibody can recognize polymorphic regions of allogeneic human leukocyte antigen molecules.

In the normal host, T cells are "trained" to recognize foreign peptides that have been expressed in the context of self-MHC molecules, and are tolerant to self-peptides. Alloreactive T cells also recognize MHC–peptide complexes through two distinct pathways: the direct allorecognition pathway, and the indirect allorecognition pathway [14,15].

Direct recognition by alloreactive T cells

In the direct pathway of allorecognition, recipient T cells recognize donor MHC–peptide complexes expressed on graft cells (see **Figure 4A**) [14–16]. T cells responding through this direct pathway are found in extremely high frequency (up to 30% of all T cells) [16–18]. As recipient T cells are "trained" during development to recognize foreign antigens expressed in the context of self-MHC, the ability to recognize a foreign MHC–peptide complex must be a manifestation of chance crossreactivity. That is, T cells specific for self-MHC plus a foreign peptide can also recognize allogeneic MHC plus an allopeptide [19].

This is not such a surprise, as the binding affinity of a TCR–MHC–peptide complex is relatively low, and there are significant similarities in overall structure between the various polymorphic MHC molecules. Notably, if the donor and recipient are fully mismatched at all MHC loci, then essentially every MHC–peptide complex expressed on graft cells is a structure that has never been "seen" before by the recipient's immune system. If the recipient's T cells recognize even a small proportion of these complexes through chance crossreactivity, then there will be a high frequency of alloreactive T cells [20].

Donor APCs (eg, dendritic cells) expressing donor MHC–peptide complexes are transplanted with the graft, and can migrate to the recipient's lymphoid organs to activate alloreactive T cells through the direct pathway [21]. These directly-primed alloreactive T cells can subsequently migrate to, and directly interact with, target cells on the graft itself, resulting in inflammation and organ damage. Experimental evidence supports the hypothesis that T cells that respond via the direct pathway account for acute cellular rejection episodes in many cases [22]. The effector pathways used by these cells to damage the graft are discussed below.

Indirect recognition by T cells

Donor graft cells can also be endocytosed by recipient APCs, with the result that donor-derived proteins can be processed into peptide

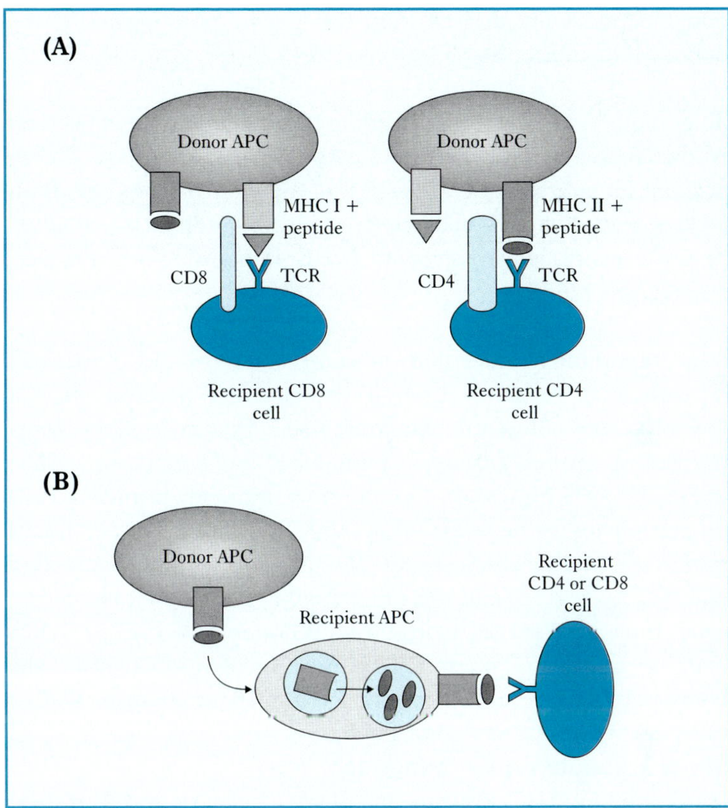

Figure 4. Alloreactive T cells recognize transplant antigens through two distinct pathways. (**A**) Recipient CD4+ and CD8+ T cells recognize and respond to donor major histocompatibility complex (MHC)–peptide complexes on graft-derived cells through the direct pathway of allorecognition. (**B**) Recipient T cells can also recognize and respond to donor-derived peptides, which are processed and presented by recipient antigen-presenting cells (APCs) on MHC molecules. This is the indirect pathway of allorecognition. TCR: T-cell receptor.

determinants and expressed on the surface of recipient APCs in the context of recipient MHC molecules [14–16,23–25]. This process is exactly the same as that which occurs with any exogenous/foreign antigen, and has been termed "indirect allorecognition" (see **Figure 4B**). In the case of transplantation antigens, the majority of donor peptides are derived from the polymorphic regions of the donor MHC molecules themselves [15,16,24,25].

The frequency of T cells responding through the indirect pathway is low compared with the direct pathway [16], and these T cells account for approximately 5%–10% of the total alloresponse. Both CD4+ and CD8+ T cells can respond to indirectly presented peptides expressed by recipient MHC II or MHC I molecules, respectively [26,27].

It is important to note that, in contrast to the direct pathway, T cells that respond through the indirect pathway do not recognize any antigen on the graft itself; they recognize donor-derived peptide antigens presented on recipient MHC molecules (see **Figure 4**). Despite this, indirectly primed T cells do participate in the rejection process, and may be preferentially important in the development of chronic allograft dysfunction [24,28–31]. As recipient APCs migrate out of the donor organ over time, they are replaced by infiltrating donor APCs [21,32], thus creating a situation in which indirect recognition may be the dominant effector pathway within the transplanted organ.

Minor transplantation antigens

In addition to MHC antigens, recipient T cells can recognize and respond to minor transplantation antigens. The clinical relevance of such antigens is illustrated by the fact that transplants between HLA-matched siblings who are not identical twins will still be rejected due to differences in expression of minor transplantation antigens. From a molecular standpoint, minor transplantation antigens can be defined as non-MHC, donor-derived peptide determinants, expressed in the context of MHC molecules common to the recipient and the donor, that are sufficiently immunogenic to induce graft rejection.

One illustrative example is the male antigen H-Y in mice (see **Figure 5**) [33–35]. Individual animals from inbred strains of mice essentially share all their genes, but males express H-Y (a series of

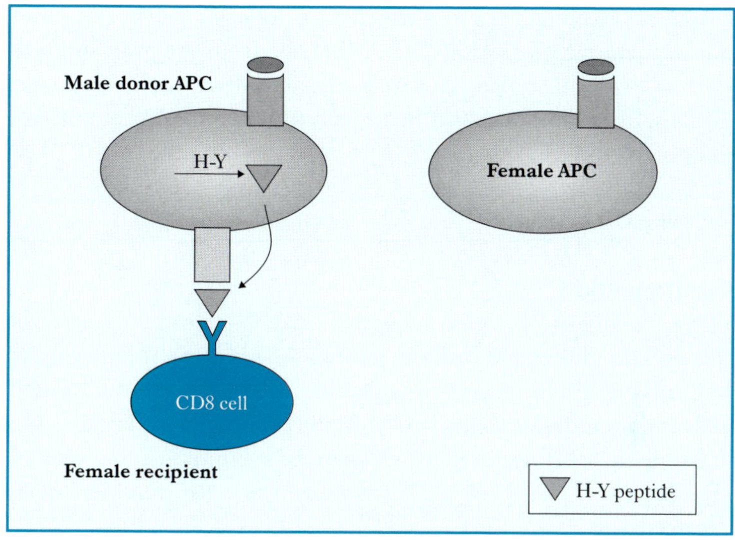

Figure 5. Representation of a minor transplantation antigen derived from the male antigen H-Y. T cells from female recipients of identical transplants derived from male donors respond to a major histocompatibility complex (MHC) class I-restricted H-Y peptide found in donor cells, but not in recipient cells. The peptide is presented in the context of MHC molecules shared between the donor and the recipient; it is only the peptide that is different between the two individuals. APC: antigen-presenting cell.

proteins specific to the male) and females do not. Female recipients can reject grafts from male mice of the same strain, and the immune response is focused towards one MHC I-restricted peptide determinant. Since the MHC I alleles are shared by both the donor and the recipient, the only immunologically relevant difference between the two animals is the peptide itself. Therefore, this immunogenic peptide represents a minor transplantation antigen. In humans, a number of minor antigens capable of initiating transplant rejection have been identified, but most are still uncharacterized.

It is important to emphasize that the initial recognition of any donor antigen by a recipient T cell is thought to occur in the secondary lymphoid organs – the lymph nodes or the spleen – and not in the graft itself [36]. Dendritic cells from the graft migrate into the secondary lymphoid organ and present an alloantigen directly, or are endocytosed by recipient APCs to present antigen indirectly to naïve T cells.

T-cell activation

Costimulation

While recipient T cells recognize MHC–peptide complexes through the direct and indirect pathways, this recognition event is not sufficient to induce full activation of the T cell. Full T-cell activation requires antigen presentation by a professional APC (ie, a dendritic cell) capable of delivering a simultaneous second signal to the T cell [7,37]. This is known as "costimulation" (see **Figure 6**).

Costimulation can be mediated through a number of molecules (several have been recently identified), but two molecules in particular appear to play an important role:

- CD28 ligand on the T cell interacts with B7-1 or B7-2 (also known as CD80 or CD86, respectively) on the APC
- CD40 ligand (CD40L, also known as CD154) on the T cell interacts with CD40 on the APC

If a T cell binds to an MHC–peptide complex in the absence of costimulation, this can potentially prevent the T cell from becoming activated, alter the T cell's function so that it becomes a regulatory or suppressor cell, or induce apoptosis of the T cell. This phenomenon is known as "costimulatory blockade".

Newly developed therapeutic agents – such as CTLA4-Ig (a chimeric molecule consisting of the common T-leukocyte antigen 4 [CTLA4] and a portion of the human immunoglobulin common region [Ig]), which blocks the CD28–B7 interaction,

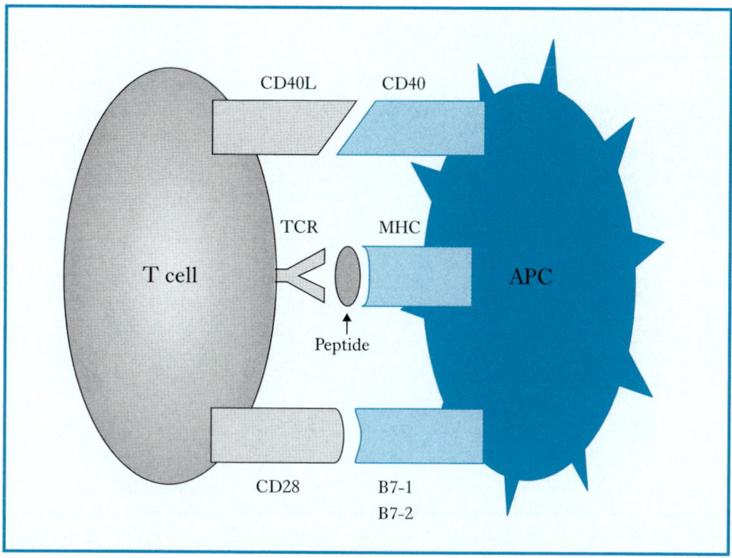

Figure 6. Costimulation is required for full activation of T cells. The best-characterized costimulatory molecules are T-cell-expressed CD28, which interacts with antigen-presenting cell (APC)-expressed B7-1 (CD80) or B7-2 (CD86), and T-cell-expressed CD40 ligand (CD40L), which interacts with APC-expressed CD40. MHC: major histocompatibility complex; TCR: T-cell receptor.

and anti-CD40L antibody, which blocks the CD40–CD40L interaction – are extremely efficient at preventing T-cell activation, and may induce true immunologic tolerance [38]. These molecules are currently being tested in clinical trials to determine their effects on prolonging human allograft survival.

If a T cell receives both a signal through the TCR and a costimulatory signal, a number of intracellular activation steps ensue (see **Figure 7**) [39–41]. A calcium flux activates the intracellular molecule calmodulin and allows it to bind to a calcium-binding protein called calcineurin (the target of the immunosuppressant drug cyclosporine A). Calcineurin activates enzymes with phosphatase activities, followed by a number of partially understood downstream reactions that lead to activation

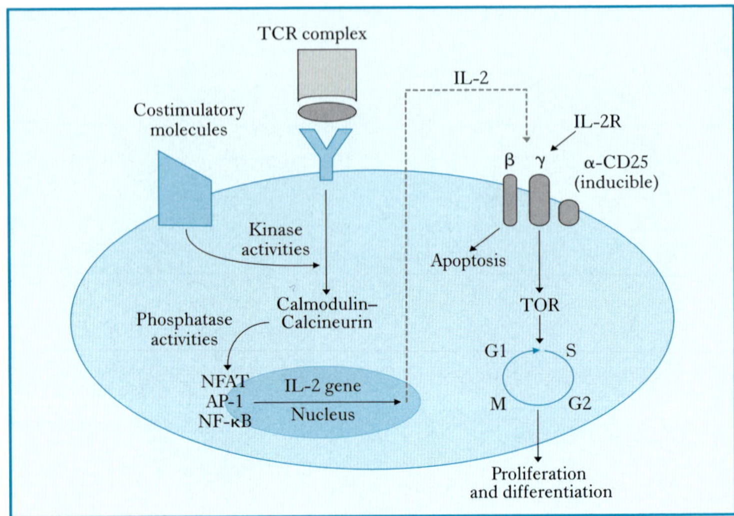

Figure 7. The intracellular signaling events associated with T-cell activation. AP: activator protein; IL: interleukin; IL-2R: interleukin-2 receptor; NFAT: nuclear factor of activated T cells; NF-κB: nuclear factor-κB; TCR: T-cell receptor; TOR: target of rapamycin.

and binding of several transcription-activating factors to the promoter of the interleukin (IL)-2 gene (among others). The molecules NFAT (nuclear factor of activated T cells), activator protein-1, and nuclear factor-κB are the best-studied transcription factors in this regard. These represent novel targets for immunosuppressive therapies aimed at controlling the alloimmune response.

The IL-2 receptor pathway

Activation of the IL-2 promoter leads to upregulation of IL-2 gene expression, followed by synthesis and release of this potent T-cell growth factor. Full T-cell activation also leads to upregulation and expression of the high-affinity γ chain of the IL-2 receptor (CD25) on the surface of the T cell (the target of anti-CD25 monoclonal antibodies). IL-2 acts in an autocrine and paracrine manner, and binds to the upregulated IL-2 receptor.

Signaling through the IL-2 receptor initiates another cascade, which is mediated, in part, through the protein "target of rapamycin" (TOR; the therapeutic target of the drug sirolimus). This results in translation of a number of new proteins, and allows the cell to progress from G1 to the S phase of the cell cycle, resulting in proliferation (the immunosuppressants azathioprine and mycophenolic acid are inhibitors of DNA synthesis, and thus inhibit T-cell activation at this stage).

T-cell differentiation

In addition to proliferation, full activation and priming of T cells results in altered expression of a variety of cell surface molecules (including upregulation of the activation marker CD44 and downregulation of the lymph node homing receptor CD62 ligand), and leads to differentiation into T cells with specific effector functions [42,43].

Effector T cells secrete cytokines and/or mediate cytotoxicity. Some T cells produce so-called "proinflammatory" type 1 cytokines, such as interferon (IFN)-γ, while others produce "anti-inflammatory" type 2 cytokines, such as IL-4, IL-10, or transforming growth factor (TGF)-β. Cytokines help to orchestrate the ensuing complex inflammatory response by regulating costimulatory molecule expression, helping to provide cell chemoattractant and activation signals, and providing a link between T-cell and B-cell immunity [5,6].

B-cell activation

B cells that recognize alloantigens through surface-bound IgM receptors also require costimulatory signals for full activation [5,6]. The costimulatory signal for B-cell activation is often delivered through CD40L, expressed on a T cell, interacting with B-cell-expressed CD40 – this illustrates the interrelationship between the cellular and humoral arms of the immune system. It has become clear that one important function of indirectly primed alloreactive T cells is to provide the helper (costimulatory) signal for B-cell activation, with subsequent induction of an alloantibody response.

Activated B cells proliferate and differentiate into antibody-secreting plasma cells through analogous intracellular signaling pathways (though distinct from those of T cells). The circulating antibody can bind to exposed alloantigens on the graft.

T-cell migration

Upon activation, T cells alter their expression of a variety of cell surface molecules, including L-selectin (the lymph node-homing receptor) and chemokine receptors, allowing them to circulate widely in the periphery [44–47].

The ability to leave the lymphoid organs is a crucial characteristic of T cells, as illustrated by the discovery that the experimental immunosuppressant FTY720 prolongs graft survival by preventing activated T cells from leaving the lymph nodes or spleen (perhaps through altering the expression of chemokine receptors).

Chemokine receptors expressed on activated T cells interact with a wide array of chemokine molecules to help facilitate recruitment to any site of inflammation, including allografts. Chemokines represent a large family of cytokines with chemoattractant properties [47–49]. These molecules can be produced by both donor graft cells and recipient immune cells, they can be constitutively produced and/or regulated by proinflammatory cytokines such as IFN-γ, and they may be upregulated by ischemia-reperfusion injury during the transplantation procedure itself [50–52].

Chemokines augment T-cell adherence to vascular endothelial cells and provide signals to enhance transmigration of T cells across vessels into the tissues. RANTES (regulated on activation, normal T-cell expressed and secreted) is one such secreted molecule that can bind to glycosaminoglycans on activated endothelium and contributes to firm attachment (stops rolling) of T cells. Release of metalloproteinases further facilitates entrance into the inflamed site.

A number of laboratories have begun to identify individual chemokines and chemokine receptors that seem to be essential for the phenotypic expression of allograft rejection. Within several years, it is anticipated that newly synthesized chemokine inhibitors will be used in clinical trials as a novel approach to prolonging allograft survival.

Effector mechanisms of graft rejection

Antibody-based effector mechanisms

Alloantibody binding to donor MHC molecules on the vascular endothelium results in a number of potential effector mechanisms [5,6]. Activation of the complement cascade can induce cell lysis, intravascular thrombosis, and organ damage (see **Figure 8A**). The resultant complement by-products (eg, C3a and C5a) also act as chemoattractants for additional inflammatory cells.

The Fc portion of the bound antibody can interact with Fc receptors expressed on macrophages and/or NK cells, resulting in macrophage (or NK-cell) activation, local production of cytokines, release of proinflammatory mediators, and subsequent destruction of the graft cells through direct cytotoxicity, among other mechanisms (see **Figure 8A**).

T-cell effector mechanisms

Primed circulating T cells will re-encounter their specific alloantigen in the graft and initiate a number of effector mechanisms. Apoptosis of donor cells is initiated through T-cell-expressed FasL interacting with Fas expressed on the graft cells [5,6]. In addition, activated effector T cells secrete perforin and granzyme B, which induce apoptosis through alternative intracellular molecular pathways (see **Figure 8B**).

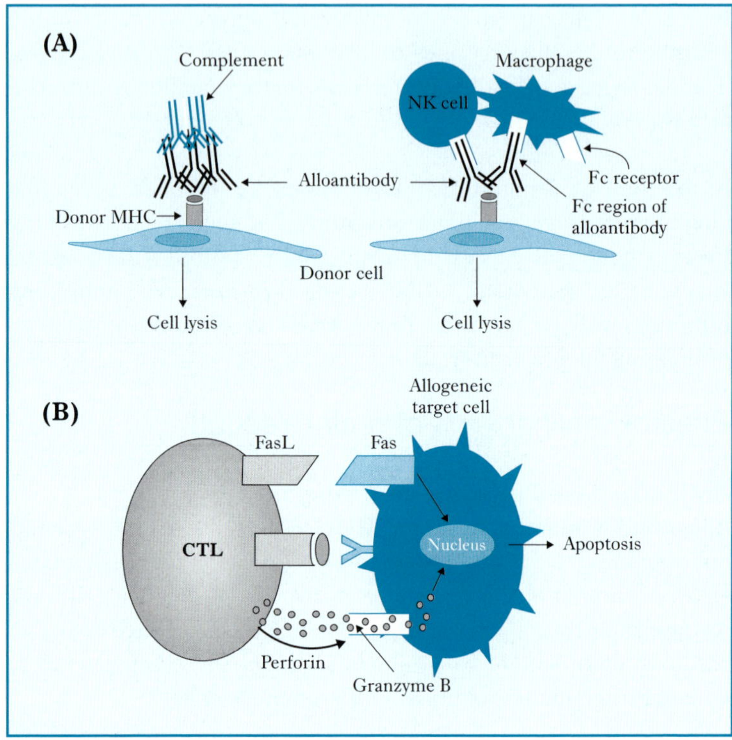

Figure 8. Effector mechanisms involved in graft destruction. (**A**) Alloantibodies can activate complement, macrophages, and natural killer (NK) cells, initiating local graft cell destruction. (**B**) Cytotoxic T cells destroy donor target cells by inducing apoptosis through Fas–Fas ligand (FasL) or perforin and granzyme B pathways. CTL: cytotoxic T lymphocyte; MHC: major histocompatibility complex.

However, cytotoxicity is not required for graft destruction [53]. As noted above, activated T cells produce proinflammatory cytokines that upregulate MHC and costimulatory molecule expression, and initiate chemoattraction and activation of mononuclear cells, particularly macrophages. T cells and macrophages can contribute to organ destruction through the co-ordinated delayed-type hypersensitivity response [54–57]. In addition, local production of nitric oxide, tumor necrosis factor-α, and TGF-β, among other proteins, can lead to direct toxicity, ischemia, and ultimately fibrosis and scarring.

Resolution

T-cell memory

Once the immune stimulus (the allograft, in the case of transplantation) has been eliminated, the inflammatory T-cell immune response resolves through activation-induced cell death, with only a residual memory T-cell pool remaining [58–60]. The resolution phase of the immune response, in which large numbers of appropriately primed T cells die, is dependent on a number of factors, including secreted cytokines (IL-2, IFN-γ, perforin, TGF-β) and cell surface molecules (CTLA4 expression on T cells).

Importantly, the residual memory T cells have lower costimulatory requirements and lower activation thresholds compared with naïve cells, enabling them to respond rapidly to a second stimulus [61–63]. While memory T cells are advantageous to the organism from an infection standpoint, such memory T-cell immunity may be particularly problematic if a second allograft is required.

B-cell memory

Similarly, B-cell memory develops as the immune response resolves. Clinicians routinely measure serum alloantibody titers using flow cytometry or standard crossmatch techniques as one measure of this memory response [2]. Those individuals with detectable antidonor alloantibodies are at high risk for the development of hyperacute or acute rejection if transplanted with an organ expressing the HLA molecule with which the specific alloantibody can interact [2].

Clinical correlates

Hyperacute rejection, immediate loss of organ function upon transplantation associated with hemorrhage, and intravascular coagulation are rarely seen in modern transplantation. The clinical syndrome of hyperacute rejection is mediated by preformed donor-reactive alloantibodies, is partially complement dependent, and is avoided through routine pretransplantation antibody crossmatching [2]. Hyperacute rejection remains a major barrier to xenotransplantation [64].

Acute rejection

Acute rejection of renal allografts most often manifests as an asymptomatic rise in serum creatinine associated with a characteristic intragraft mononuclear cell infiltrate within the first 3–6 months posttransplantation [2]. Experimental evidence suggests that T cells that respond through the direct pathway of allorecognition are likely to be the major pathologic mediators of acute rejection [22].

T cells that respond to minor transplantation antigens and alloantibodies missed in a pretransplant crossmatch, or alloantibodies that develop posttransplantation, clearly contribute to acute rejection in some situations [2]. Detection of C4d (another complement activation by-product) deposition in renal allografts is the molecular standard for diagnosing antibody-mediated renal allograft rejection [75].

Chronic allograft dysfunction

Chronic allograft dysfunction (chronic rejection) can be defined as a chronic deterioration of graft function that cannot be explained by other known processes [2]. For renal allografts, it is commonly characterized by hypertension and proteinuria, and has a characteristic histology of interstitial fibrosis, vasculopathy, and glomerulosclerosis.

The pathogenesis of this entity is poorly understood, but both immune and nonimmune mechanisms contribute. While T cells that respond directly to donor APCs are associated with acute cellular rejection, it has been hypothesized that T cells that respond through the indirect pathway may be the predominant mediators of chronic rejection (see **Figure 9**) [24,31,55,65–69].

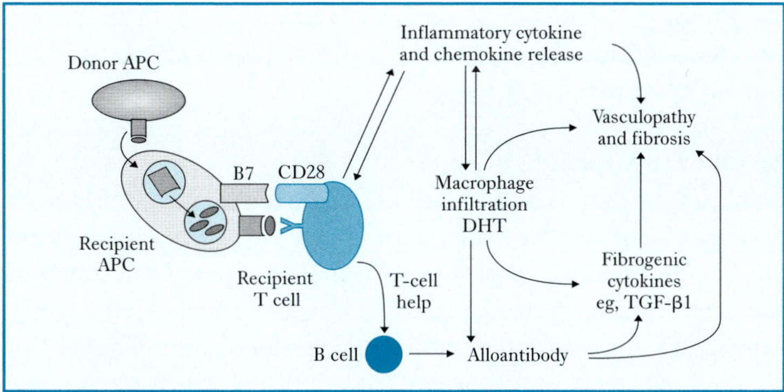

Figure 9. Proposed immune effector mechanisms that result in chronic allograft dysfunction following indirect allorecognition. APC: antigen-presenting cell; DTH: delayed-type hypersensitivity; TGF: transforming growth factor.

Inflammation

As noted above, donor APCs that are transplanted with the organ rapidly leave the graft and are replaced by infiltrating recipient APCs. Under such conditions, donor-derived peptides can be processed and presented by recipient APCs within the graft itself, permitting specific interactions between indirectly primed T cells and their antigenic targets in the transplanted organ. These T cells cannot directly mediate destruction of donor cells through cognate interactions, but can induce nonspecific inflammation through cytokine production and macrophage-mediated effector functions (ie, delayed-type hypersensitivity).

Posttransplant alloantibody responses

Indirectly primed T cells can provide helper costimulatory signals for induction of a posttransplant alloantibody response [28,70]. Furthermore, the presence and development of alloantibodies posttransplant correlates with the development of chronic allograft dysfunction [29,30,71,72]. Adoptive transfer of allospecific antibodies into immunodeficient recipients of allografts can reproduce transplant vasculopathy in animal models, providing further support for the hypothesis that alloantibodies contribute to the pathologic phenotype of chronic rejection [73,74]. The specific effector mechanisms involved in the development of these lesions remain an active area of research.

Nonimmune factors

Nonimmune factors also contribute to the development of fibrosis and vasculopathy in both animals and humans [29,30,71,72]. Brain death of the donor and prolonged ischemia-reperfusion injury of the graft are thought to enhance the immunogenicity of the donor organ, and are associated with a higher risk for development of chronic allograft dysfunction. In addition, the size of the transplanted organ, hypertension, drug toxicity (eg, from chronic cyclosporine use), and a variety of other factors are associated with the development of chronic graft dysfunction. Clearly, the pathogenic mechanisms that result in chronic rejection/organ dysfunction are still poorly understood, and remain a prominent area of research in transplantation immunobiology.

Conclusion

Organ transplantation results in a potent alloreactive humoral and cellular immune response capable of rapidly destroying a donor graft. It is hoped that a thorough comprehension of the complexities, redundancies, and interrelationships between the various components of this pathogenic alloimmune response will provide new clues to designing therapies aimed at prolonging the survival of transplants in humans.

References

1. Rosenberg A, Singer A. Cellular basis of skin allograft rejection: an in vivo model of immune-mediated tissue destruction. *Annu Rev Immunol* 1992;10:333–58.
2. Suthanthiran M, Strom T. Renal transplantation. *N Engl J Med* 1994;331:365–76.
3. Silvers WK, Billingham RE. The tissue typing and lymphocyte problems in transplantation immunity. *Med Clin North Am* 1965;49:1661–74.
4. Rosenberg A. Skin allograft rejection. In: Coligan J, Kruisbeek A, Margulies D et al., editors. *Current Protocols in Immunology*. Bethesda: John Wiley and Sons, Inc, 1991:4.4.1–4.4.9.
5. Delves PJ, Roitt IM. The immune system. First of two parts. *N Engl J Med* 2000; 343:37–49.

6. Delves PJ, Roitt IM. The immune system. Second of two parts. *N Engl J Med* 2000; 343:108–17.
7. Sayegh MH, Turka LA. The role of T-cell costimulatory activation pathways in transplant rejection. *N Engl J Med* 1998;338:1813–21.
8. Demant P. H-2 gene complex and its role in alloimmune reactions. *Transplant Rev* 1973;15:162–200.
9. Klein J, Sato A. The HLA system. Second of two parts. *N Engl J Med* 2000;343:782–6.
10. Sumitran-Holgersson S. HLA-specific alloantibodies and renal graft outcome. *Nephrol Dial Transplant* 2001;16:897–904.
11. Bohmig GA, Exner M, Watschinger B et al. Acute humoral renal allograft rejection. *Curr Opin Urol* 2002;12:95–9.
12. Baid S, Saidman SL, Tolkoff-Rubin N et al. Managing the highly sensitized transplant recipient and B cell tolerance. *Curr Opin Immunol* 2001;13:577–81.
13. Sheldon S, Dyer PA. HLA antigen mismatching and HLA-specific antibodies in heart transplantation: review of a single center experience. The Manchester Wythenshawe Heart Transplant Team. *Transplant Proc* 1992;24:2438.
14. Gould DS, Auchincloss H Jr. Direct and indirect recognition: the role of MHC antigens in graft rejection. *Immunol Today* 1999;20:77–82.
15. Auchincloss H Jr, Sultan H. Antigen processing and presentation in transplantation. *Curr Opin Immunol* 1996;8:681–7.
16. Benichou G, Valujskikh A, Heeger PS. Contributions of direct and indirect T cell alloreactivity during allograft rejection in mice. *J Immunol* 1999;162:352–8.
17. Ashwell J, Chen C, Schwartz R. High frequency and nonrandom distribution of alloreactivity in T cell clones selected for recognition of foreign antigen in association with self class II molecules. *J Immunol* 1986;136:389–95.
18. Heeger PS, Greenspan NS, Kuhlenschmidt S et al. Pretransplant frequency of donor-specific, IFN-gamma-producing lymphocytes is a manifestation of immunologic memory and correlates with the risk of posttransplant rejection episodes. *J Immunol* 1999;163:2267–75.
19. Reiser JB, Darnault C, Guimezanes A et al. Crystal structure of a T cell receptor bound to an allogeneic MHC molecule. *Nat Immunol* 2000;1:291–7.
20. Matesic D, Lehmann PV, Heeger PS. High-resolution characterization of cytokine-producing alloreactivity in naive and allograft-primed mice. *Transplantation* 1998; 65:906–14.
21. Saiki T, Ezaki T, Ogawa M et al. In vivo roles of donor and host dendritic cells in allogeneic immune response: cluster formation with host proliferating T cells. *J Leukoc Biol* 2001;69:705–12.
22. Pietra BA, Wiseman A, Bolwerk A et al. CD4 T cell-mediated cardiac allograft rejection requires donor but not host MHC class II. *J Clin Invest* 2000;106:1003–10.
23. Auchincloss H Jr, Lee R, Shea S et al. The role of "indirect" recognition in initiating rejection of skin grafts from major histocompatibility complex class II-deficient mice. *Proc Natl Acad Sci USA* 1993;90:3373–7.
24. Vella JP, Spadafora-Ferreira M, Murphy B et al. Indirect allorecognition of major histocompatibility complex allopeptides in human renal transplant recipients with chronic graft dysfunction. *Transplantation* 1997;64:795–800.
25. Watschinger B, Gallon L, Carpenter CB et al. Mechanisms of allo-recognition. Recognition by in vivo-primed T cells of specific major histocompatibility complex polymorphisms presented as peptides by responder antigen-presenting cells. *Transplantation* 1994;57:572–6.
26. Valujskikh A, Hartig C, Heeger PS. Indirectly primed CD8+ T cells are a prominent component of the allogeneic T-cell repertoire after skin graft rejection in mice. *Transplantation* 2001;71:418–21.

27. Matzinger P, Bevan MJ. Induction of H-2-restricted cytotoxic T cells: in vivo induction has the appearance of being unrestricted. *Cell Immunol* 1977;33:92–100.
28. Vella JP, Magee C, Vos L et al. Cellular and humoral mechanisms of vascularized allograft rejection induced by indirect recognition of donor MHC allopeptides. *Transplantation* 1999;67:1523–32.
29. Womer KL, Vella JP, Sayegh MH. Chronic allograft dysfunction: mechanisms and new approaches to therapy. *Semin Nephrol* 2000;20:126–47.
30. Knoflach A, Chandraker A, Sayegh MH. Chronic rejection from bedside to bench: role of T cells. *Ann Transplant* 1997;2:53–60.
31. Sayegh MH, Carpenter CB. Role of indirect allorecognition in allograft rejection. *Int Rev Immunol* 1996;13:221–9.
32. Saiki T, Ezaki T, Ogawa M et al. Trafficking of host- and donor-derived dendritic cells in rat cardiac transplantation: allosensitization in the spleen and hepatic nodes. *Transplantation* 2001;71:1806–15.
33. Scott DM, Ehrmann IE, Ellis PS et al. Why do some females reject males? The molecular basis for male-specific graft rejection. *J Mol Med* 1997;75:103–14.
34. Greenfield A, Scott D, Pennisi D et al. An H-YDb epitope is encoded by a novel mouse Y chromosome gene. *Nat Genet* 1996;14:474–8.
35. Silvers WK, Billingham RE, Sanford BH. The H-Y transplantation antigen: a Y-linked or sex-influenced factor? *Nature* 1968;220:401–3.
36. Lakkis FG, Arakelov A, Konieczny BT et al. Immunologic "ignorance" of vascularized organ transplants in the absence of secondary lymphoid tissue. *Nat Med* 2000;6:686–8.
37. Yamada A, Salama AD, Sayegh MH. The role of novel T cell costimulatory pathways in autoimmunity and transplantation. *J Am Soc Nephrol* 2002;13:559–75.
38. Larsen CP, Elwood ET, Alexander DZ et al. Long-term acceptance of skin and cardiac allografts after blocking CD40 and CD28 pathways. *Nature* 1996;381:434–8.
39. Krensky AM. T cells in autoimmunity and allograft rejection. *Kidney Int Suppl* 1994; 44:S50–S56.
40. Halloran PF. Molecular mechanisms of new immunosuppressants. *Clin Transplant* 1996;10:118–23.
41. Healy JI, Goodnow CC. Positive versus negative signaling by lymphocyte antigen receptors. *Annu Rev Immunol* 1998;16:645–70.
42. Reinhardt RL, Khoruts A, Merica R et al. Visualizing the generation of memory CD4 T cells in the whole body. *Nature* 2001;410:101–5.
43. Masopust D, Vezys V, Marzo AL et al. Preferential localization of effector memory cells in nonlymphoid tissue. *Science* 2001;291:2413–7.
44. von Andrian UH, Mackay CR. T-cell function and migration. Two sides of the same coin. *N Engl J Med* 2000;343:1020–34.
45. Sallusto F, Lenig D, Forster R et al. Two subsets of memory T lymphocytes with distinct homing potentials and effector functions. *Nature* 1999;401:708–12.
46. Springer TA. Traffic signals for lymphocyte recirculation and leukocyte emigration: the multistep paradigm. *Cell* 1994;76:301–14.
47. Westermann J, Engelhardt B, Hoffmann JC. Migration of T cells in vivo: molecular mechanisms and clinical implications. *Ann Intern Med* 2001;135:279–95.
48. Luster AD. The role of chemokines in linking innate and adaptive immunity. *Curr Opin Immunol* 2002;14:129–35.
49. Kunkel EJ, Butcher EC. Chemokines and the tissue-specific migration of lymphocytes. *Immunity* 2002;16:1–4.
50. Kapoor A, Morita K, Engeman TM et al. Intragraft expression of chemokine gene occurs early during acute rejection of allogeneic cardiac grafts. *Transplant Proc* 2000;32:793–5.

51. Kapoor A, Morita K, Engeman TM et al. Early expression of interferon-gamma inducible protein 10 and monokine induced by interferon-gamma in cardiac allografts is mediated by CD8+ T cells. *Transplantation* 2000;69:1147–55.
52. Fairchild RL, VanBuskirk AM, Kondo T et al. Expression of chemokine genes during rejection and long-term acceptance of cardiac allografts. *Transplantation* 1997;63:1807–12.
53. VanBuskirk AM, Wakely ME, Orosz CG. Acute rejection of cardiac allografts by noncytolytic CD4(+) T cell populations. *Transplantation* 1996;62:300–2.
54. Coito AJ, Binder J, Brown LF et al. Anti-TNF-alpha treatment down-regulates the expression of fibronectin and decreases cellular infiltration of cardiac allografts in rats. *J Immunol* 1995;154:2949–58.
55. Valujskikh A, Matesic D, Gilliam A et al. T cells reactive to a single immunodominant self-restricted allopeptide induce skin graft rejection in mice. *J Clin Invest* 1998;101: 1398–407.
56. Russell ME. Macrophages and transplant arteriosclerosis: known and novel molecules. *J Heart Lung Transplant* 1995;14:S111–S115.
57. Nagano H, Libby P, Taylor MK et al. Coronary arteriosclerosis after T-cell-mediated injury in transplanted mouse hearts: role of interferon-gamma. *Am J Pathol* 1998; 152:1187–97.
58. Wagener ME, Konieczny BT, Dai Z et al. Alloantigen-driven T cell death mediated by Fas ligand and tumor necrosis factor-alpha is not essential for the induction of allograft acceptance. *Transplantation* 2000;69:2428–32.
59. Hassan AT, Dai Z, Konieczny BT et al. Regulation of alloantigen-mediated T-cell proliferation by endogenous interferon-gamma: implications for long-term allograft acceptance. *Transplantation* 1999;68:124–9.
60. Dai Z, Konieczny BT, Baddoura FK et al. Impaired alloantigen-mediated T cell apoptosis and failure to induce long-term allograft survival in IL-2-deficient mice. *J Immunol* 1998,161.1659–63.
61. Viola A, Lanzavecchia A. T cell activation determined by T cell receptor number and tunable thresholds. *Science* 1996;273:104–6.
62. Pihlgren M, Dubois PM, Tomkowiak M et al. Resting memory CD8+ T cells are hyperreactive to antigenic challenge in vitro. *J Exp Med* 1996;184:2141–51.
63. London CA, Lodge MP, Abbas AK. Functional responses and costimulator dependence of memory CD4+ T cells. *J Immunol* 2000;164:265–72.
64. Auchincloss H Jr, Sachs DH. Xenogeneic transplantation. *Annu Rev Immunol* 1998; 16:433–70.
65. Hornick PI, Mason PD, Baker RJ et al. Significant frequencies of T cells with indirect anti-donor specificity in heart graft recipients with chronic rejection. *Circulation* 2000;101:2405–10.
66. Coelho V, Spadafora-Ferreira M, Marrero I et al. Evidence of indirect allorecognition in long-term human renal transplantation. *Clin Immunol* 1999;90:220–9.
67. Womer KL, Sayegh MH, Auchincloss H Jr. Involvement of the direct and indirect pathways of allorecognition in tolerance induction. *Philos Trans R Soc Lond B Biol Sci* 2001;356:639–47.
68. Lee RS, Yamada K, Houser SL et al. Indirect recognition of allopeptides promotes the development of cardiac allograft vasculopathy. *Proc Natl Acad Sci USA* 2001;98:3276–81.
69. Chen W, Murphy B, Waaga AM et al. Mechanisms of indirect allorecognition in graft rejection: class II MHC allopeptide-specific T cell clones transfer delayed-type hypersensitivity responses in vivo. *Transplantation* 1996;62:705–10.
70. Steele DJ, Laufer TM, Smiley ST et al. Two levels of help for B cell alloantibody production. *J Exp Med* 1996;183:699–703.
71. Libby P, Pober JS. Chronic rejection. *Immunity* 2001;14:387–97.

72. Orosz CG, Pelletier RP. Chronic remodeling pathology in grafts. *Curr Opin Immunol* 1997;9:676–80.
73. Russell PS, Chase CM, Winn HJ et al. Coronary atherosclerosis in transplanted mouse hearts. II. Importance of humoral immunity. *J Immunol* 1994;152:5135–41.
74. Russell PS, Chase CM, Winn HJ et al. Coronary atherosclerosis in transplanted mouse hearts. III. Effects of recipient treatment with a monoclonal antibody to interferon-gamma. *Transplantation* 1994;57:1367–71.
75. Collins AB, Schneeberger EE, Pascual MA et al. Complement activation in acute humoral renal allograft rejection: diagnostic significance of C4d deposits in peritubular capillaries. *J Amer Soc Nephrol* 1999; 10:2208–14.

3

Immunosuppressive drug therapy

Anthony J Langone & J Harold Helderman

Introduction

The discovery and routine use of cyclosporine in the early 1980s led to immediate benefits for renal transplant recipients, manifested primarily by improved 1-year renal allograft survival rates. In addition, it has become apparent that long-term graft survival rates have also increased [1]. This improvement may be caused by a generalized rise in the total immunosuppression delivered to the patient.

Immunosuppressive protocols that aggressively attempt to prevent acute rejection episodes make strategic sense, as the number, severity, and timing of acute rejection episodes correlate with the development of chronic allograft nephropathy (CAN) [2,3]. Death with a functioning graft and CAN are the most common reasons for renal transplant failure.

The bane of the transplant community, CAN is the yoke that prevents truly spectacular graft half-lives. Unfortunately, a uniform etiology of CAN escapes current understanding. Both immune injury, possibly mediated by donor-specific antibodies [4], and nonimmune factors, such as hypertension and chronic ischemia/vasoconstriction, may contribute to the pathophysiology of CAN.

Infections have also been shown to play a role in the pathogenesis of CAN. Aggressive prophylaxis against viral pathogens, especially cytomegalovirus, may contribute to the longer half-lives of renal allografts that have been reported in recent years. Paradoxically, certain immunosuppressants (eg, calcineurin inhibitors; see below) have been implicated in the pathogenesis of CAN. As the causes of CAN become better understood, immunosuppressant protocols may be tailored to avoid the development of CAN in patients at risk.

Induction therapy

The incidence of acute rejection is greatest in the first few months after transplantation, when the body attempts to accommodate the foreign organ. Thus, the delivery of immunosuppression is typically highest during the perioperative period. An immunosuppressive strategy known as "induction therapy" may be employed, where the early posttransplant protocol includes antibodies against specific or multiple antigenic targets.

The benefits of using such induction antibodies to reduce the risk of early acute rejection must be weighed against the cost of these agents, and the potentially increased risk of over-immunosuppression, manifested by infection or malignancy. While there has been a slow but progressive trend toward increasing use of induction agents in the US (approximately 50% of transplant centers in the US utilize induction protocols), the large majority of transplant centers worldwide avoid induction therapy with antibodies. Some centers use antibody induction therapy only in selected patients who are perceived to be at high risk for allograft rejection. In addition, these antibodies are often used in patients with delayed graft function in order to postpone the initiation of treatment with potentially nephrotoxic calcineurin inhibitors [5].

Monoclonal antibodies

Anti-CD25 antibodies

Interleukin (IL)-2 plays a critical role in the immune response. This cytokine binds to a specific receptor (CD25) on the surface of activated T cells, and stimulates a cascade of events that result in cell cycle progression from the G1 (growth) phase to the S (synthesis) phase (see Chapter 2). Since the mid-1990s, two monoclonal anti-CD25 antibodies have been developed against the α subunit of the IL-2 receptor.

One agent, basiliximab (Simulect), is a chimeric antibody consisting of approximately 70% human immunoglobulin (Ig) and 30% mouse Ig. The murine component represents the variable sections of the heavy and light chains. The antibody specifically binds, with high affinity, to the α chain of the IL-2 receptor on activated T cells. Inactive lymphocytes do not express the IL-2 receptor, and are therefore largely unaffected.

The second anti-CD25 antibody, daclizumab (Zenapax), is humanized with >90% human and 10% mouse Ig. It also binds to the α chain of the IL-2 receptor, but with less affinity than basiliximab, as only the hypervariable regions of the heavy and light chains are murine. Both of these antibodies have long half-lives, and are well tolerated with few, if any, side effects. Anaphylactic reactions are exceedingly rare [6], and neutralizing antimouse antibodies are seldom encountered.

When compared with placebo, treatment with either basiliximab [7] or daclizumab [8] has been associated with a lower rate of early acute rejection, but long-term outcomes remain to be determined. Basiliximab is typically administered intraoperatively, and again on postoperative day 4. Although daclizumab was originally marketed to be delivered in five doses over 10 weeks, one- [9] and two-dose [10] regimens have proven to be effective in reducing rejection rates.

OKT3

The monoclonal antibody OKT3 (Orthoclone Muromonab-CD3) has been engineered to target the CD3 complex of mature T cells. Binding to the CD3 complex results in endocytosis of its constituent peptides, leading to marked impairment of T-cell activation and proliferation.

Prior to causing T-cell inactivation, OKT3 stimulates T cells to make a variety of cytokines that are responsible for a "first-dose effect", manifested by fever, headache, myalgia, and rigor. Occasionally, this cytokine-release syndrome is manifested by hypotension or pulmonary edema. These symptoms can be mitigated if OKT3 is administered while the patient is intubated, sedated, and paralyzed during the initial transplant operation. The risk of pulmonary edema can be minimized by ensuring that the patient is within 5% of his or her dry weight prior to treatment. An experimental, humanized form of the drug may have equivalent efficacy with minimal first-dose effects.

Neutralizing antimurine antibodies commonly develop during or after administration of OKT3, and may limit the drug's efficacy, especially in patients receiving multiple courses of therapy. Routine monitoring of CD3 counts or antimouse antibody titers is performed to ensure drug efficacy. OKT3 is highly effective in reversing ongoing episodes of acute rejection, even in patients who have been resistant to treatment with other agents [11]. However, many centers now prefer to use either anti-CD25 agents or polyclonal agents (see below) for induction therapy, reserving OKT3 for the treatment of acute rejection, if needed.

Polyclonal antibodies

Polyclonal antibodies directed against multiple antigenic targets are commonly used for induction therapy. Currently, two polyclonal agents are commercially available: antithymocyte globulin (ATG) derived from rabbit (Thymoglobulin), and ATG derived from horse (ATGAM).

When compared with no antibody induction therapy, both agents are associated with lower rates of early acute rejection and improved long-term graft survival [12,13]. Compared with anti-CD25 antibodies or OKT3, disadvantages of these agents include a requirement for central venous infusion (or very prolonged peripheral infusion) to prevent venous sclerosis, and the need for 7–14 days of therapy. However, a recent study suggests that a 3-day course of rabbit ATG is as effective as a 7-day course [14]. Moreover, daily monitoring of CD3 counts may allow substantial dose reductions [15].

First-dose side effects can occur with polyclonal agents, but tend to be milder than those observed with OKT3. Both equine and rabbit ATG can cause transient leukopenia and/or thrombocytopenia, which often necessitate dose adjustments. Use of large doses or prolonged courses of therapy are occasionally complicated by serum sickness.

Which induction antibody?

Head-to-head comparisons of the available agents have yielded mixed results. One study indicated that rabbit ATG is superior to equine ATG for induction therapy [16]. A comparison of OKT3 with equine ATG showed a trend toward better patient and graft survival with OKT3 at significantly less cost [17]. A randomized trial comparing basiliximab with equine ATG found no difference in quality-adjusted patient survival, but concluded that ATG was significantly more expensive [18]. Newer regimens that utilize smaller total doses of ATG (three or four-dose induction regimens) while providing the same level of immunosuppressive efficacy might reduce the aforementioned total cost differences between agents.

In patients who are highly sensitized, anti-CD25 antibodies do not offer as much protection against acute rejection as polyclonal agents [19]. Thus, the choice of induction therapy is individualized and center-specific. One strategy adopted at some centers has been to use anti-CD25 antibodies in patients at lower risk for allograft rejection, and polyclonal agents or OKT3 in highly sensitized patients and others perceived to be at high risk for rejection.

Maintenance therapy

Unfortunately, only a small number of transplant recipients completely accommodate their allograft such as to allow total cessation of immunosuppression. Because it is currently impossible to identify such individuals, lifelong immunosuppression is the current standard of practice to prevent acute rejection and graft loss in all kidney transplant recipients. Although individuals who completely stop their immunosuppression (usually as a result of noncompliance) may appear to be functionally tolerant of their grafts for years, an immunomodulating virus (such as a flu virus) may upregulate the recipient's immune system at some future time point, and lead to late and devastating rejection.

Maintenance immunosuppressive therapy represents a delicate balance between providing enough immunosuppression to prevent rejection and avoiding excessive immunosuppression, which can increase the risk of infection and malignancy. Most centers employ multiple (typically three) drug regimens in order to minimize the toxicity of any single agent and to inhibit the immune response via separate, but additive or synergistic, mechanisms.

Calcineurin inhibitors

Cyclosporine preparations

Since the introduction of cyclosporine, calcineurin inhibitors have become the cornerstone of most maintenance immunosuppression protocols. After binding to cytosolic proteins known as immunophilins, these agents inhibit the phosphatase calcineurin, which is essential in the signal transduction pathway that ultimately leads to transcription of the gene for IL-2.

Cyclosporine binds to the immunophilin cyclophilin and inhibits generation of IL-2. Other mechanisms of cyclosporine action have also been proposed [20], including enhanced transcription of transforming growth factor-β. Cyclosporine has revolutionized the field of organ transplantation by significantly improving short-term allograft outcomes when compared with patients treated with azathioprine and corticosteroids. Unfortunately, cyclosporine is a critical-dose drug with large intra- and interindividual variations in bioavailability, and a narrow window between efficacious and toxic doses. Acute and chronic nephrotoxicity are the most concerning side effects.

The pathophysiology of cyclosporine-mediated renal vasoconstriction remains incompletely understood. Possible mechanisms include activation of the sympathetic nervous system, activation of the renin–angiotensin system, nitric oxide inhibition, upregulation of endothelin, and corruption of the prostaglandin system [21]. Other side effects of cyclosporine include hirsutism, gingival hyperplasia, tremor, hyperlipidemia, hypertension, glucose intolerance, and hyperkalemia.

The first cyclosporine formulation (Sandimmune) was an oil-based compound that relied on the patient's bile production for absorption. A newer cyclosporine preparation, Neoral, is a microemulsion that eliminates the need for bile production, and has reduced intrapatient variability and improved bioavailability. Use of the microemulsion formulation has reduced the risk of CAN and improved long-term allograft survival [22].

The ability to estimate a patient's total exposure to cyclosporine is considered essential in maintaining efficacy and minimizing toxicity. Cyclosporine bioavailability, as estimated by the pharmacologic "area under the curve" (AUC), is a sensitive predictor of acute rejection and graft survival [23]. However, measurements of AUCs are cumbersome and impractical for routine patient management. Traditionally, trough blood concentrations have been utilized to estimate total exposure to a drug. Compared with Sandimmune, use of Neoral results in a stronger correlation between the measured trough blood concentration and total drug exposure as estimated by the AUC.

Two studies have suggested that measuring the serum cyclosporine level 2 hours after dose ingestion correlates significantly better with the AUC than a trough level [24,25]. The 2-hour cyclosporine level, known as the "C_2 level", holds promise for better long-term graft outcomes with cyclosporine use.

A number of generic alternatives to both the oil-based and microemulsion formulations of cyclosporine are now available, and represent a special concern with this critical-dose drug. In the US, the Food and Drug Administration only loosely defines bioequivalence between generic drugs and the original compounds they wish to emulate. Thus, high rates of inter- and intrapatient variability can be expected when the cyclosporine formulation is changed. A reasonable approach to this issue consists of educating patients to notify their physician of formulation changes, monitoring drug levels in the near-term to determine the dosage required to obtain target serum concentrations, and guiding patients to pharmacies whose generic predilections are known and consistent.

Tacrolimus

A newer calcineurin inhibitor, tacrolimus (FK-506, Prograf), binds to a different immunophilin (FK-binding protein), but has a mechanism of action similar to that of cyclosporine. In most randomized prospective trials that have compared tacrolimus with cyclosporine, tacrolimus has been associated with a lower rate of early acute rejection, without an appreciable influence on long-term patient or graft survival [26–28]. Most studies have compared tacrolimus with the original oil-based cyclosporine formulation, and there are few data comparing tacrolimus with the microemulsion formula. Tacrolimus has been touted as a "rescue agent" capable of reversing acute rejection episodes that are resistant to cyclosporine-based therapy [29].

Despite a similar mechanism of action, the toxicity profile of tacrolimus differs from that of cyclosporine: both drugs are potentially nephrotoxic; tacrolimus is not associated with hirsutism or gingival hyperplasia, but is occasionally a cause of alopecia; neurotoxicity (tremors, seizures, and encephalopathy) is generally more common and severe with tacrolimus therapy; and tacrolimus is clearly more diabetogenic than cyclosporine, and is associated with a higher rate of new-onset diabetes mellitus following transplantation [30,31].

Corticosteroids

Although corticosteroids (eg, prednisone) have been used to prevent and treat allograft rejection for several decades, their mechanism of action remains incompletely understood. Steroids induce the transcription of inhibitory factor-κB proteins, which prevent the transcription of genes encoding a number of proinflammatory cytokines. In addition, steroids exert nonspecific anti-inflammatory actions that inhibit monocyte migration into areas of inflammation.

Deleterious side effects associated with chronic steroid use include bone loss, cushingoid features, obesity, susceptibility to hematoma, hypertension, hyperlipidemia, diabetes mellitus, and cataract formation. In general, there has been a trend toward using lower doses of these agents in order to minimize side effects, and based on the premise that calcineurin inhibitors and other modern immunosuppressants are "steroid-sparing". Moreover, there has been a resurgence of interest in steroid avoidance and steroid withdrawal protocols.

In the cyclosporine–azathioprine era (1983–1995), even patients at low immunologic risk experienced an unacceptably high rate (>30%) of acute rejection when steroids were withdrawn [32]. More importantly, a number of studies from that era indicated that steroid withdrawal increased the long-term risk of allograft loss [33]. It appears that steroids might sensitize lymphocytes, such that late withdrawal may, in theory, be worse than complete avoidance [34]. In addition, many of the side effects of steroids, such as osteopenia, occur early and irreparably with steroid exposure [35]. Thus, more recent interest has focused on using some of the newer immunosuppressant agents in protocols that employ very early withdrawal of steroids [36] or complete avoidance of these agents [37].

Antimetabolites

The antimetabolites azathioprine (Imuran) and mycophenolate mofetil (MMF; CellCept) exert their action by blocking DNA synthesis.

Azathioprine

Azathioprine, a purine analogue, inhibits both the *de novo* and salvage pathways of nucleotide synthesis, thereby interrupting the S phase of the cell cycle. Historically, azathioprine was the first immunosuppressive agent used in an effort to prevent allograft rejection in human kidney transplant recipients. The drug was originally used as a monotherapy, but results improved substantially when corticosteroids were added.

Most of the side effects of azathioprine are the result of its suppression of rapidly dividing cells. Leukopenia and thrombocytopenia are dose-related side effects that typically respond to downward dose adjustments. The recent introduction of generic azathioprine has raised less controversy than the generic cyclosporines because *de novo* use of azathioprine has largely been supplanted by MMF.

Mycophenolate mofetil

MMF has been increasingly used in multidrug immunosuppression protocols since the mid-1990s. A prodrug, MMF is rapidly hydrolyzed within the gastrointestinal tract to the active molecule, mycophenolic acid. Similar to azathioprine, MMF interrupts the S phase of the cell cycle. However, the drug specifically inhibits the enzyme inosine monophosphate dehydrogenase, which is rate limiting in the *de novo* pathway of purine synthesis. Because lymphocytes are relatively deficient in enzymes of the salvage pathway for purine synthesis, MMF is more specific to the inhibition of T and B cells than azathioprine [38]. MMF also inhibits the glycosylation of proteins that may prevent some of the structural changes characteristic of CAN.

Three pivotal studies showed that the use of MMF in combination with cyclosporine and steroids resulted in a significant reduction in the incidence of acute rejection when compared with azathioprine or placebo (also in combination with cyclosporine and steroids) [39–41]. These individual studies were not statistically powered to show a benefit of MMF on graft survival.

However, a pooled analysis of the three studies [42] and a subsequent registry analysis [43] suggest that use of MMF increases long-term graft survival.

The most common dose-related side effects of MMF are diarrhea, nausea, vomiting, and bone marrow suppression. Because mycophenolic acid is excreted by the kidneys, some transplant physicians empirically lower the dose of MMF in the presence of renal insufficiency.

TOR inhibitors

Sirolimus (rapamycin, Rapamune) is a macrocyclic compound with potent immunosuppressive properties. It binds to the same immunophilin, FK-binding protein, as tacrolimus. The sirolimus–FK-binding protein complex has no effect on calcineurin, and instead inhibits the mammalian target of rapamycin (mTOR), a cytosolic enzyme that regulates growth and proliferation of lymphocytes during the G1 phase of the cell cycle.

When used in combination with cyclosporine and steroids, sirolimus has been proven to be safe and efficacious in reducing acute rejection rates in clinical trials [44]. Common dose-dependent side effects include thrombocytopenia and hyperlipidemia. Idiosyncratic reactions include apthous ulcer formation, interstitial pneumonitis, and rash. The anti-proliferative effects of the drug may be responsible for impaired wound healing, including a relatively high incidence of lymphoceles [45].

The use of sirolimus with cyclosporine appears to be a potent and synergistic combination, which may safely allow steroid withdrawal [46]. Although tacrolimus and sirolimus bind to the same immunophilin, the abundance of intracellular FK-binding protein allows the two drugs to be used in combination with excellent efficacy [47,48]. Sirolimus may facilitate withdrawal or avoidance of calcineurin inhibitors [49–51]. Sirolimus may also

Side effect	Cyclosporine	Tacrolimus	Prednisone	AZA	MMF	Sirolimus
Acne	0	0	↑↑	0	0	0
Alopecia	0	↑↑	0	0	0	0
Anemia	0	0	0	0	0	↑↑
Diabetes	↑	↑↑↑	↑↑	0	0	0
Gastrointestinal	0	↑↑	0	0	↑↑↑	↑
Gingival hyperplasia	↑↑↑	0	0	0	0	0
Hematoma	0	0	↑↑	0	0	0
Hirsutism	↑↑↑	0	0	0	0	0
HUS/TTP	↑↑↑	↑↑	0	0	0	↑
Hyperlipidemia	↑↑	0	↑	0	0	↑↑↑
Hypertension	↑↑	↑	↑	0	0	0
Insomnia	0	0	↑↑	0	0	0
Leukopenia	0	0	0	↑↑	↑↑↑	0
Neurologic	↑	↑↑↑	↑	0	0	0
Obesity	0	0	↑↑↑	0	0	0
Malignancy	↑	↑	↓	↑↑↑	↑	↓↓↓
Osteoporosis	0	0	↑↑↑	0	0	0
Thrombocytopenia	0	0	0	↑↑	↑	↑↑↑

Table 1. Side effects of maintenance immunosuppressants. AZA: azathioprine; HUS: hemolytic uremic syndrome; MMF: mycophenolate mofetil; TTP: thrombotic thrombocytopenic purpura; ↑: increased effect; ↓: decreased effect; 0: no change.

prevent CAN by inhibiting the expression of growth factor mRNAs [52], or by inhibiting the proliferation of smooth muscle cells involved in the characteristic vasculopathy. Patients with established CAN or calcineurin inhibitor toxicity may also benefit from conversion to rapamycin treatment [53]. Finally, sirolimus has important antineoplastic properties [54], and may prove to be a drug that can be safely continued to prevent allograft rejection in transplant recipients who have developed a malignancy.

Conclusion

The days of "one protocol fits all" for kidney transplant recipients are long gone. The advantages, nuances, and side effects of each immunosuppressant (see **Table 1**) should lead the transplant professional to tailor a regimen specific to each patient.

During the past decade, the development of several new immunosuppressants has increased the number of drug combinations that can be used to individualize immunosuppression, and ongoing trials continue to test various combinations of agents. Ironically, as more potent drugs with novel mechanisms of action are developed, some of the immunosuppressants once considered to be the cornerstones of therapy will be abandoned in an effort to eliminate their toxicities and prolong the survival of kidney transplant patients and their allografts.

References

1. Hariharan S, Johnson CP, Bresnahan BA et al. Improved graft survival after renal transplantation in the United States, 1988 to 1996. *N Engl J Med* 2000;342:605–12.
2. Basadonna G, Matas A, Gillingham K et al. Early versus late acute renal allograft rejection: Impact on chronic rejection. *Transplantation* 1993;55:993–5.
3. van Saase J, van der Woude F, Thorogood J et al. The relation between acute vascular and interstitial renal allograft rejection and subsequent chronic rejection. *Transplantation* 1995;59:1280–5.
4. Pelletier RP, Hennessy PK, Adams PW et al. Clinical significance of MHC-reactive alloantibodies that develop after kidney or kidney–pancreas transplantation. *Am J Transplant* 2002;2:134–41.
5. Lange H, Muller TF, Ebel H et al. Immediate and long-term results of ATG induction therapy for delayed graft function compared to conventional therapy for immediate graft function. *Transpl Int* 1999;12:2–9.

6. Novartis Pharmaceutical Canada Inc. Product monograph: Simulect (basiliximab), September 1, 2000.
7. Nashan B, Moore R, Amlot P et al. Randomised trial of basiliximab versus placebo for control of acute cellular rejection in renal allograft recipients. CHIB 201 International Study Group. *Lancet* 1997;350:1193–8.
8. Vincenti F, Kirkman R, Light S et al. Interleukin-2 receptor blockade with daclizumab to prevent acute rejection in renal transplantation. Daclizumab Triple Therapy Study Group. *N Engl J Med* 1998;338:161–5.
9. Ahsan N, Holman MJ, Jarowenko MV et al. Limited dose monoclonal IL-2R antibody induction protocol after primary kidney transplantation. *Am J Transplant* 2002;2:568–73.
10. ter Meulen CG, Baan CC, Hene RJ et al. Two doses of daclizumab are sufficient for prolonged interleukin-2Ralpha chain blockade. *Transplantation* 2001;72:1709–10.
11. Norman DJ, Kahana L, Stuart FP Jr et al. A randomized clinical trial of induction therapy with OKT3 in kidney transplantation. *Transplantation* 1993;55:44–50.
12. Szczech LA, Berlin JA, Aradhye S et al. Effect of anti-lymphocyte induction on renal allograft survival: a meta-analysis. *J Am Soc Nephrol* 1997;8:1771–7.
13. Belitsky P, MacDonald AS, Lawen J et al. Use of rabbit anti-thymocyte globulin for induction immunosuppression in high-risk kidney transplant recipients. *Transplant Proc* 1997;29(Suppl 7A):16S–17S.
14. Agha IA, Rueda J, Alvarez A et al. Short-course induction immunosuppression with thymoglobulin for renal transplant recipients. *Transplantation* 2002;73:473–5.
15. Peddi VR, Bryant M, Roy-Chaudhury P et al. Safety, efficacy, and cost analysis of thymoglobulin induction therapy with intermittent dosing based on CD3+ lymphocyte counts in kidney and kidney–pancreas transplant recipients. *Transplantation* 2002;73:1514–8.
16. Brennan DC, Flavin K, Lowell J et al. A randomized, double-blinded comparison of Thymoglobulin versus Atgam for induction immunosuppression therapy in adult renal transplant recipients. *Transplantation* 1999;67:1011–8.
17. Kumar MS, Cahill K, Kumar AM et al. ATGAM versus OKT3 induction therapy in cadaveric kidney transplantation: patient and graft survival, CD3 subset, infection, and cost analysis. *Transplant Proc* 1998;30:1351–2.
18. Polsky D, Weinfurt KP, Kaplan B et al. An economic and quality-of-life assessment of basiliximab vs. antithymocyte globulin immunoprophylaxis in renal transplantation. *Nephrol Dial Transplant* 2001;16:1028–33.
19. Mariat C, Afiani A, Alamartine E et al. A pilot study comparing basiliximab and anti-thymocyte globulin as induction therapy in sensitized renal allograft recipients. *Transplant Proc* 2001;33:3192–3.
20. Halloran PF. Mechanism of action of the calcineurin inhibitors. *Transplant Proc* 2001;33:3067–9.
21. McNally PG, Feehally J. Pathophysiology of cyclosporin A nephrotoxicity: experimental and clinical observation. *Nephrol Dial Transplant* 1992;7:791–804.
22. Meier-Kriesche HU, Kaplan B. Cyclosporine microemulsion and tacrolimus are associated with decreased chronic allograft failure and improved long-term graft survival as compared with Sandimmune. *Am J Transplant* 2002;2:100–4.
23. Kahan BD, Welsh M, Rutzky LP. Challenges in cyclosporine therapy: the role of therapeutic monitoring by area under the curve monitoring. *Ther Drug Monit* 1995;17:621–4.
24. Mahalati K, Belitsky P, Sketris I et al. Neoral monitoring by modified sparse sampling area under the concentration–time curve: its relationship to acute rejection and cyclosporine nephrotoxicity early after kidney transplantation. *Transplantation* 1999;68:55–62.

25. Primmett DR, Levine M, Kovarik JM et al. Cyclosporine monitoring in patients with renal transplants: two- or three-point methods that estimate area under the curve are superior to trough levels in predicting drug exposure. *Ther Drug Monit* 1998;20:276–83.
26. Vincenti F, Laskow DA, Neylan JF et al. One-year follow-up of an open label trial of FK506 for primary kidney transplantation. A report of the U.S. Multicenter FK506 Kidney Transplant Group. *Transplantation* 1996;61:1576–81.
27. Knoll GA, Bell RC. Tacrolimus versus cyclosporine for immunosuppression in renal transplantation: meta-analysis of randomised trials. *BMJ* 1999;318:1104–7.
28. Pirsch JD, Miller J, Deierhoi MH et al. A comparison of tacrolimus (FK506) and cyclosporine for immunosuppression after cadaveric renal transplantation. FK506 Kidney Transplant Study Group. *Transplantation* 1997;63:977–83.
29. Jordan ML, Shapiro R, Vivas CA et al. FK506 "rescue" for resistant rejection of renal allografts under primary cyclosporine immunosuppression. *Transplantation* 1994; 57:860–5.
30. Panz VR, Bonegio R, Raal FJ et al. Diabetogenic effect of tacrolimus in South African patients undergoing kidney transplantation. *Transplantation* 2002;73:587–90.
31. Maes BD, Kuypers D, Messiaen T et al. Posttransplantation diabetes mellitus in FK-506-treated renal transplant recipients: analysis of incidence and risk factors. *Transplantation* 2001;72:1655–61.
32. Hricik DE, Seliga RM, Fleming-Brooks S et al. Determinants of long-term allograft function following steroid withdrawal in renal transplant recipients. *Clin Transplant* 1995;9:419–23.
33. Hricik DE. Steroid-free immunosuppression in kidney transplantation: an editorial review. *Am J Transplant* 2002;2:19–24.
34. Almawi WY, Hess DA, Assi JW et al. Pretreatment with glucocorticoids enhances T-cell effector: possible implication for immune rebound accompanying glucocorticoid withdrawal. *Cell Transplant* 1999;8:637–47.
35. Keogh A, Macdonald P, Harvison A et al. Initial steroid-free versus steroid-based maintenance therapy and steroid withdrawal after heart transplantation: two views of the steroid question. *J Heart Lung Transplant* 1992;11:421–7.
36. Matas AJ, Ramcharan T, Paraskevas S et al. Rapid discontinuation of steroids in living donor kidney transplantation: a pilot study. *Am J Transplant* 2001;1:278–83.
37. Birkeland SA. Steroid-free immunosuppression in renal transplantation: a long-term follow-up of 100 consecutive patients. *Transplantation* 2001;71:1089–90.
38. Morris RE, Hoyt EG, Murphy MP et al. Mycophenolic acid morpholinoethylester (RS-61443) is a new immunosuppressant that prevents and halts heart allograft rejection by selective inhibition of T- and B-cell purine synthesis. *Transplant Proc* 1990;22:1659–62.
39. The Tricontinental Mycophenolate Mofetil Renal Transplantation Study Group. A blinded, randomized clinical trial of mycophenolate mofetil for the prevention of acute rejection in cadaveric renal transplantation. *Transplantation* 1996;61:1029–37.
40. European Mycophenolate Mofetil Cooperative Study Group. Placebo-controlled study of mycophenolate mofetil combined with cyclosporine and corticosteroids for the prevention of acute rejection. *Lancet* 1995;345:1321–5.
41. Sollinger HW. Mycophenolate mofetil for the prevention of acute rejection in primary cadaveric renal allograft recipients. US Renal Transplant Mycophenolate Mofetil Study Group. *Transplantation* 1995;60:225–32.
42. Halloran P, Mathew T, Tomlanovich S et al. Mycophenolate mofetil in renal allograft recipients: A pooled efficacy analysis of three randomized, double-blind, clinical studies in prevention of rejection. The International Mycophenolate Mofetil Renal Transplant Study Group. *Transplantation* 1997;63:39–47.

43. Ojo AO, Meier-Kriesche HU, Hanson JA et al. Mycophenolate mofetil reduces late renal allograft loss independent of acute rejection. *Transplantation* 2000;69:2405–9.
44. MacDonald AS. A worldwide, phase III, randomized, controlled, safety and efficacy study of a sirolimus/cyclosporine regimen for prevention of acute rejection in recipients of primary mismatched renal allografts. *Transplantation* 2001;71:271–80.
45. Langer RM, Kahan BD. Incidence, therapy, and consequences of lymphocoele after sirolimue–cyclosporine–prednisone immunosuppression in renal transplant recipients. *Transplantation* 2002;74:804–8.
46. Mahalati K, Kahan BD. A pilot study of steroid withdrawal from kidney transplant recipients on sirolimus–cyclosporine A combination therapy. *Transplant Proc* 2001;33:3232–3.
47. Hartwig T, Pridohl O, Witzigmann H et al. Low-dose sirolimus and tacrolimus in kidney transplantation: first results of a single-center experience. *Transplant Proc* 2001;33:3226–8.
48. Lawen J, Keough-Ryan T, Clase C et al. Sirolimus and low-dose tacrolimus with antibody induction in kidney transplantation: preliminary results of a pilot study. *Transplant Proc* 2001;33:3223–5.
49. Groth CG, Backman L, Morales JM et al. Sirolimus (rapamycin)-based therapy in human renal transplantation: similar efficacy and different toxicity compared with cyclosporine. Sirolimus European Renal Transplant Study Group. *Transplantation* 1999;67:1036–42.
50. Kreis H, Cisterne JM, Land W et al. Sirolimus in association with mycophenolate mofetil induction for the prevention of acute graft rejection in renal allograft recipients. *Transplantation* 2000;69:1252–60.
51. Johnson RW, Kreis H, Oberbauer R et al. Sirolimus allows early cyclosporine withdrawal in renal transplantation resulting in improved renal function and lower blood pressure. *Transplantation* 2001;72:777–86.
52. Oliveira JG, Xavier P, Sampaio SM et al. Compared to mycophenolate mofetil, rapamycin induces significant changes on growth factors and growth factor receptors in the early days post-kidney transplantation. *Transplantation* 2002;73:915–20.
53. Diekmann F, Waiser J, Fritsche L et al. Conversion to rapamycin in renal allograft recipients with biopsy-proven calcineurin inhibitor-induced nephrotoxicity. *Transplant Proc* 2001;33:3234–5.
54. Luan FL, Hojo M, Maluccio M et al. Rapamycin blocks tumor progression: unlinking immunosuppression from antitumor efficacy. *Transplantation* 2002;73:1565–72.

4

Evaluation of kidney transplant recipients and donors

Moro O Salifu & Mariana S Markell

Introduction

The science of renal transplantation is exemplified by the Confucian saying, "A journey of a thousand miles begins with the first step." The choice of recipient and donor are the first steps that influence the ultimate survival of the allograft.

It is clear that chronic rejection is the end result of both immunologic and nonimmunologic factors [1]. It is also clear that donor and recipient characteristics modify these factors, and thus play a role in long-term kidney transplant outcome. This chapter reviews the latest recommendations for evaluating and selecting kidney transplant recipients and living donors.

Recipient evaluation

Initial evaluation

The American Society of Transplantation (AST) issued clinical practice guidelines for the evaluation of renal transplant recipients [2]. Within these guidelines, it is stated that, "Evaluation begins when the patient is referred for transplantation." The routes by which patients come to evaluation for transplantation are varied, and include self-referral, or referral by a primary physician, another type of primary care provider, or subspecialist (such as a nephrologist).

Contraindications to kidney transplantation
Malignancy
Chronic infection
• HIV[a]
• Active hepatitis B
• Tuberculosis
• Peritonitis
• Chronic skin infection
• Chronic osteomyelitis
Untreated severe coronary artery disease
Severe peripheral vascular disease
Cirrhosis of the liver
Chronic obstructive pulmonary disease
Noncompliance
Psychiatric illness
Active substance abuse
Lack of insurance or inability to pay for medication

Table 1. Contraindications to kidney transplantation. [a]Human immunodeficiency virus (HIV) is currently a contraindication to transplantation in most centers; however, HIV-infected patients who are free of opportunistic infections, with a stable undetectable viral load, and CD4 lymphocyte count >300/mm^3 may be considered for renal transplantation.

Contraindications to kidney transplantation

Although relatively few absolute contraindications to renal transplantation exist, their presence should be determined as soon as possible to avoid false expectations and unnecessary expense. These include: inability to pay for the transplant procedure or immunosuppressive medications (ie, patients who are ineligible for insurance or whose insurance company will not reimburse for transplantation), certain malignancies treated within the past 2–5 years, HIV infection (see below for detail), irreversible cardiac disease that would pose a substantial operative risk (eg, heart failure or coronary artery disease), active substance abuse, evidence of severe psychiatric disease, and active chronic infection (see **Table 1**).

Cancer

Patients with a history of cancer and those with treatable infection or cardiac disease can be advised to follow-up with specialty providers and return for re-evaluation. Most centers require at least 2–5 years after a cancer-free diagnosis before a patient can be listed for cadaveric transplantation or be a candidate to receive living donor kidney transplantation (see **Table 2**).

Transplantation of the kidney alone is not recommended for patients with multiple myeloma (because of frequent recurrence posttransplant) or for those with localized liver cancer (unless a concomitant liver transplant is to be attempted). Combined bone marrow kidney transplantation for multiple myeloma is largely experimental [3]. Patients with basal cell skin cancer do not require a waiting period.

Infection

The goal of screening for infection is to detect and eradicate infections that may be worsened by immunosuppressive therapy. Since it is not possible to screen for all infections, the pretransplant evaluation is generally tailored towards commonly encountered infections, notably HIV, active hepatitis B, tuberculosis (TB), peritonitis (in patients receiving peritoneal dialysis), and skin infections related to diabetes.

HIV

Although the prevalence of HIV positivity in the dialysis population ranges from 0.3% to 2.6% [4,5], 88% of transplant centers surveyed in the US did not consider cadaver kidney transplantation

Type of cancer	Waiting time (years)	Comments
Renal cell carcinoma		
<5 cm	2	Incidental tumors <5 cm found at nephrectomy require no waiting
>5 cm	5	
Wilm's tumor	2	Patients with Deny–Drash[a] syndrome should undergo bilateral nephrectomy
Bladder	2	*In situ* or noninvasive papilloma requires no waiting
Anogenital malignancies	No data	No data
Uterine cancer		
Localized cervical	2–5	No data on invasive cervical cancer, but probably >5 years
Uterine body	2	
Testicular carcinoma	2	
Thyroid carcinoma	2	
Kaposi's/other sarcomas	2	HHV-8 serology should be determined for high-risk patients (Middle Eastern, African)
Breast cancer, invasive	5	2 years for localized cancers
Colorectal carcinoma	5	2 years for Duke's A or B1; 5 years for Duke's B2, C1, or C2
Prostate cancer	2	No waiting for localized disease
Liver cancer	Contraindicated	May be considered for combined liver–kidney transplant, if localized
Active multiple myeloma	Contraindicated	MGU is not an absolute contraindication
Lymphoma/leukemia	2	EBV-negative serology identifies those at risk for PTLD
Skin cancers		<5 years if *in situ* or thin melanoma
Melanoma	5	
Squamous cell	2	
Basal cell	None	
Lung cancer	2	

Table 2. Minimum cancer-free waiting times for kidney transplant recipients. [a]Autosomal recessive mutation in Wilm's tumor suppressor gene (*WT1*). EBV: Epstein–Barr virus; HHV-8: human herpes virus-8; MGU: monoclonal gammopathy of undetermined significance; PTLD: posttransplant lymphoproliferative disease.

in this population, while 91% did not consider living donor kidney transplantation [6]. Experimental evidence regarding transplantation in HIV-infected individuals is still lacking. In one retrospective analysis of HIV-positive cadaver kidney transplant recipients prior to highly active antiretroviral therapy (HAART), using the US Renal Data System (USRDS), the 3-year graft and patient survival were 53% and 83%, respectively, compared with 73% and 88% for HIV-negative recipients [7].

Until evidence accumulates, most centers would reject HIV-infected patients for transplantation. However, HIV-infected patients who are free of opportunistic infections, compliant with HAART, with stable undetectable viral load, and CD4 lymphocyte counts >300/mm^3 may be considered for renal transplantation [8].

Tuberculosis

Although asymptomatic in most cases, TB is a commonly encountered infection in the dialysis population, who appear to be more susceptible to TB infection than the general population. Immunosuppression may reactivate TB, which tends to be aggressive and disseminated [9,10]. While purified protein derivative positivity in dialysis patients is up to 9% [11], the prevalence of active TB posttransplant in the western world ranges between 0.4%–1.7% [9,12], and higher in developing nations [10,12].

Thus, the AST Clinical Practice Guidelines recommend that patients with active TB receive “adequate treatment”, and that patients with a recent positive tuberculin skin test or chest x-ray suspicious for quiescent TB receive TB prophylaxis prior to transplantation [2].

Peritonitis

Peritonitis occurs in up to 13% of peritoneal dialysis patients within 90 days posttransplant [13]. Successful posttransplant treatment of peritonitis has been reported in children [14]. Risk factors for this complication include frequent episodes of peritonitis pretransplant, peritonitis due to *Staphylococcus aureus*, and male gender. The risk of peritonitis is significantly reduced if peritoneal dialysis catheters are removed within 6 days of transplantation [15].

A safe interval between resolution of peritonitis and transplantation has not been established in peritoneal dialysis patients. Given that transplantation in peritoneal dialysis patients is generally safe [15], adequate treatment of peritonitis and documentation of eradication of infection prior to transplantation is a prudent strategy.

Hepatitis

Hepatitis B or C history, followed by serologic validation, should be obtained prior to accepting candidates for transplantation. Administration of the hepatitis B vaccine should be considered in patients who test negative for hepatitis B, in accordance with established guidelines for vaccination in dialysis patients [16]. Patients who are hepatitis B surface antigen (HBsAg)-positive have an increased risk for death following transplantation. The risk of death is greatest with concomitant hepatitis C infection or active hepatitis B infection (hepatitis B envelope antigen [HBeAg]-positive) [17].

Most centers do not exclude HBsAg-positive patients from transplantation if there is no evidence of active disease on liver biopsy, and if they are HBeAg-negative [18,19]. Unlike interferon, lamivudine is a safe and effective antiviral hepatitis B treatment that can be used both before and after kidney transplantation. Lamivudine therapy commenced at transplantation should prevent early posttransplant reactivation of hepatitis B, and subsequent progression to cirrhosis and late liver failure. This pre-emptive therapy should also eradicate early liver failure from fibrosing cholestatic hepatitis [20].

As there is no consensus on the long-term effects of hepatitis C on renal or patient survival, the presence of hepatitis C antibody is not a contraindication to transplantation. Many centers follow a similar protocol for hepatitis C as for hepatitis B, recommending liver biopsy if there is evidence of active liver disease, and making case by case decisions regarding transplantation [18,19].

Cytomegalovirus

Serologic validation of cytomegalovirus (CMV) positivity should be performed in both recipients and donors prior to transplantation, in order to determine the risk of true disease and need for prophylaxis (acyclovir, ganciclovir, valacyclovir, and intravenous gammaglobulin). If both donor and recipient are negative for CMV antibody, the incidence of CMV disease in the recipient is only 5% [20], and thus prophylaxis is not recommended. If the donor is positive and recipient negative for CMV antibody, the incidence of CMV disease is as high as 50%–75% [20,21], necessitating prophylaxis. An intermediate risk of 25%–40% is present when the recipient is CMV antibody-positive and the donor is either positive or negative; in this case, prophylaxis is discretional [20].

Prophylaxis is also indicated if the recipient undergoes antilymphocyte antibody therapy, and either the recipient or donor is CMV antibody-positive [20]

Other latent infections

Though electively performed, serologic screening for other chronic viral infections – such as Epstein–Barr virus (EBV), human herpes virus type 8 (HHV-8), Varicella–Zoster virus (VZV), herpes simplex virus (HSV), and human T-lymphotropic virus type 1 (HTLV-1) – may yield useful information regarding posttransplant prophylaxis or surveillance [2]. Seronegative EBV recipients, particularly pediatric patients, are at high risk for EBV infection transmitted via donor kidney posttranplant, which may increase the risk of posttransplant lymphoproliferative disease (PTLD). Although evidence is lacking, seronegative recipients may benefit from antiviral prophylaxis, such as acyclovir or ganciclovir posttransplant. Seropositive HHV-8 (in high-risk patients, such as those from the Middle East and Africa) and HTLV-1 recipients are at increased risk for Kaposi's sarcoma and PTLD, respectively. As no prophylactic antiviral regimen has been demonstrated for these recipients, close surveillance for unexplained weight loss, nonspecific symptoms, and lymphadenopathy may identify those with PTLD who can be salvaged with immunosuppression dose reduction or chemotherapy. Seropositive VZV, HSV, and toxoplasmosis identifies those at risk for reactivation and treatment, rather than prophylaxis, when true disease occurs posttransplant. Seropositive VDRL recipients should be treated prior to transplantation.

Preventive maintenance

As part of preventive maintenance, all candidates should be reviewed to ensure the recommended vaccinations [16] have been administered for both adults and children. Moreover, as pre- and posttransplant periodontal disease are very much correlated [22], the diagnosis and treatment of periodontal disease prior to transplantation may decrease the incidence of gingival hyperplasia.

Cardiovascular disease

Cardiovascular disease is probably the most commonly encountered issue when evaluating candidates for transplantation. Cardiovascular disease accounts for almost half of all deaths that occur within the first 30 days of transplantation. The AST Clinical Practice Guidelines suggest that patients with a history of ischemic heart disease, or who are symptomatic for ischemic heart disease, should undergo cardiac catheterization to delineate the extent of coronary disease amenable to surgical repair prior to transplantation [2].

Asymptomatic patients or those without a history of ischemic heart disease can be selected for noninvasive cardiac testing based on clinical criteria. Clinical parameters linked to posttransplant ischemic heart disease include age >50 years, diabetes, and an abnormal electrocardiogram [23,24].

Peripheral vascular disease

Peripheral vascular disease (PVD) is a further concern when evaluating patients for transplantation. In one report, the incidence of PVD in patients with end-stage renal disease was 4.2% at 5 years and 5.9% at 10 years [9,11], and was particularly high in those with diabetes mellitus.

Atherosclerotic aorto-iliac disease can make transplantation technically challenging, if not impossible. It is recommended that patients with physical or symptomatic evidence of PVD be screened by Doppler ultrasound or other noninvasive imaging studies (eg, helical computerized tomography or magnetic resonance angiography); reconstruction is usually successful [25,26]. Patients with a history of transient ischemic attack or carotid bruit should undergo Doppler imaging or angiography if clinically indicated to detect significant occlusive disease prior to transplantation.

Genitourinary dysfunction

Finally, issues regarding genitourinary dysfunction must be addressed prior to the placement of a new kidney. Although voiding cystourethrograms are no longer routinely performed due to a low yield of significant anomalies, this procedure should be considered in certain circumstances (eg, congenital abnormalities, pediatric recipients, and patients with a prior history of voiding problems).

Pretransplant native kidney nephrectomy is not recommended, except in cases of extremely large polycystic kidneys, chronic parenchymal infection, persistent severe nephrotic syndrome, or refractory hypertension despite adequate medical therapy.

Summary of pretransplant evaluations

Table 3 summarizes routine and elective pretransplant evaluations. A survey of 154 European transplant centers undertaken in 2000 revealed wide variation among the actual screening procedures performed in potential kidney transplant recipients [27]. Of note, 39% of centers routinely ordered voiding cystourethrograms on all patients, 44% routinely conducted echocardiography, and 16% performed peripheral Doppler ultrasound studies. Only 21% of the centers routinely ordered tuberculin skin testing, and 47% tested for syphilis. Almost all (>90%) agreed that hepatitis B, CMV, and hepatitis C serologies, chest x-ray, and an electrocardiogram were necessary.

Routine	Elective
Full history and physical exam	Voiding cystourethrogram
Coagulation profile	Exercise treadmill
Blood typing	Echocardiogram
Serology for HBsAg, HBsAb, HCV antibody, VDRL, HIV, HSV, CMV	Coronary angiogram
Pelvic exam and Pap smear	EBV, VZV, HSV, HTLV-1 toxoplasmosis, lipid profile, PPD
Chest radiograph	Prostate-specific antigen
Electrocardiography	Vascular studies
Psychosocial	Gastrointestinal studies
Complete blood count and chemistry	Mammogram
Tissue-typing and panel-reactive antibody (cadaveric recipients)	Electrophoresis

Table 3. Pretransplant evaluations for kidney transplant recipients. CMV: cytomegalovirus; EBV: Epstein–Barr virus; HBsAb: hepatitis B surface antibody; HBsAg: hepatitis B surface antigen; HCV: hepatitis C virus; HIV: human immunodeficiency virus; HSV: herpes simplex virus; HTLV-1: human T-lymphotropic virus type 1; Pap: Papanicolaou; PPD: purified protein derivative; VDRL: Venereal Disease Research Laboratory test; VZV: Varicella–Zoster virus.

Rescreening of listed candidates

The recommendations for rescreening a patient who was initially deemed acceptable for transplantation have not been standardized. Unfortunately, in many regions, there may be a delay of several years between a patient's initial placement on the cadaveric transplant waiting list and the actual transplant procedure itself.

In 2001, a survey of 192 transplant centers undertaken by the Clinical Practice Guidelines Committee of the AST found that 59% of centers rescreened diabetic patients for coronary artery disease, and 53% rescreened patients with documented coronary artery disease, irrespective of the presence of diabetes mellitus [28]. The majority of these centers (79%) rescreened patients on an annual basis. The methods used varied widely and included nuclear perfusion studies, dobutamine echocardiography, and coronary angiography.

In the same survey, 80% of centers rescreened patients for hepatitis viruses and 52% rescreened for "other infectious diseases". Cancer screening was variable, with many programs leaving the decision to the local nephrologist. It was recommended that annual follow-up appointments be scheduled via routine scheduling or program-initiated telephone contact. High-risk patients (those who are older, obese, or diabetic) should be monitored "more frequently" (no specific recommendations were given) [28].

The most serious problem in the follow-up of wait-listed patients was a lack of uniformity in communication between the dialysis unit and the transplant center regarding changes in a patient's health status [28]. Most centers expected the dialysis unit to apprise them of clinical events, and 20% expected the patient to do so, with 17% reporting no policy about such communications.

One impediment to communication is the large number of patients on waiting lists, which necessitates a huge work-load in collecting follow-up data. It is estimated that, for a center with a waiting list of 500 patients, approximately 40 patient contacts/ month are required in order to update the list appropriately. The obvious recommendation is to create ways of decreasing waiting time and list length. Until that happens, meticulous follow-up is imperative to avoid assigning kidneys to patients who are no longer eligible for transplantation.

Other recommendations

Postoperative cardiopulmonary risk may be reduced by cessation of smoking, maintenance of optimal weight, moderate exercise as tolerated, dietary counseling, and adequate control of diabetes, hypertension, and heart disease.

Body weight

Although there is no recommendation for an ideal preoperative body weight, in one study, a body mass index (BMI) of <30 kg/m^2 compared with >30 kg/m^2 was associated with fewer superficial wound breakdowns (4% vs. 14%, $P < 0.01$) and complete wound dehiscence (0% vs. 3%, $P < 0.01$). Wound infections also tended to be more frequent in obese recipients (15% vs. 8%, $P = 0.11$). There were no significant differences between the two groups with respect to operative duration, postoperative complications, hospitalization, delayed graft function, or acute rejection episodes. Five-year actuarial survival rates were comparable between the two groups with respect to graft survival (83% vs. 84%) and patient survival (91% vs. 91%) [29].

Cancer detection

For early cancer detection, age-specific screening recommendations exist for the detection of prostate, breast, cervical, and colorectal cancer [30], and should be followed for all patients referred for listing. Men >40 years old should have digital rectal examination, and those >50 years old should have both digital rectal examination and measurement of prostate-specific antigen. Women 20–65 years old should have a Papanicolaou smear test, and those >40 years should have mammography.

Colorectal screening should be performed for all individuals >50 years using stool occult blood testing, digital rectal examination, and/or direct visualization of the lower gastrointestinal tract via colonoscopy. Colonoscopy is mandatory in cases of iron-deficiency anemia.

Allosensitization

Allosensitization may be reduced by avoiding blood transfusions, especially in patients with a high percentage of panel-reactive antibodies. Immunization for health maintenance should be administered as indicated, with the understanding that patients who receive dialysis may require extra doses or increased strength of vaccines in order to achieve immunity, particularly when vaccinating against hepatitis B.

Substance abuse and noncompliance

Substance abuse and noncompliance should be addressed. Individuals with known or suspected chemical dependence should be referred for substance-abuse counseling. In patients with chemical dependence, documentation of successful cessation for at least 6 months is recommended by the AST Clinical Practice Guidelines [2].

Patients with suspected or documented noncompliance with dialysis or medications may be at risk for noncompliance during the posttransplant period. A frank discussion with the patient regarding the need for improved compliance and documentation of an attempt by the patient may be warranted prior to proceeding with transplantation.

Some patients exhibit noncompliance behavior during dialysis as a manifestation of depression, or frustration with the constraints imposed by the dialytic lifestyle. If depression or anxiety disorder is suspected, referral for psychiatric evaluation is mandatory, as high-dose steroid hormones administered in the early transplant period may exacerbate either condition, with negative consequences.

Special considerations

Pre-emptive transplantation

Patients with chronic kidney disease may be referred for transplantation when creatinine clearance is <20 mL/min, allowing them to accrue time on the waiting list for a cadaver transplant, prior to the initiation of dialysis. If a living donor is available, planning for pre-emptive transplantation may be conducted prior to the development of symptomatic uremia. Pre-emptive living donor transplantation has been reported to result in better outcomes than living donor transplants performed following the initiation of dialysis [31].

Potential living donors may be biologically related, emotionally related, or, at some centers, purely altruistic with no tie to the recipient. The timing of pre-emptive transplantation is variable, but the goal is to maximize the period during which the patient's own kidneys function, while avoiding the complications of advanced uremia. Frequent visits to a nephrologist, including careful review of symptoms, physical examination, and laboratory testing, are imperative during the pretransplant period. If medically indicated, dialysis should never be delayed while awaiting transplantation.

Age limits

In the US, there are currently no recommendations for an upper age limit to transplantation. The age at which hemodialysis is initiated is shifting upwards, with an estimated 9% of patients >65 years old on the waiting list for cadaver transplants [32]. Data from the USRDS suggest that kidney transplant recipients aged 60–74 years old have better transplant survival than age-matched controls on the waiting list [33]. Because this group of patients are at increased risk for cardiovascular death, they require more frequent follow-up while on the waiting list.

Although 5% of pediatric kidney transplants are performed on children <2 years old [32], overall graft survival is better when a target weight of 15 kg is reached [34], unless an emergency transplant is required because of lack of access to dialysis.

Evaluation of living kidney donors

Because of the potential for better long-term graft survival, a lower incidence of acute rejection, and improved quality of life, living kidney donation should be pursued for all candidates for kidney transplantation. It is imperative to ensure, however, that the decision to donate is voluntary, and without any financial compensation. The evaluation process should be friendly, cost-effective, and expedited to allow donors to move quickly through the process.

Living kidney donation is generally safe, with mortality estimated at 0.03% and morbidity at 0.23% [23]. The development of laparoscopic nephrectomy techniques (see Chapter 5) has decreased the length of hospital stay [35]. The result is less time lost from work with less potential for lost income, improved direct and indirect costs related to hospital stay, and increased donation rates [35].

In one single-center experience, data were obtained for 464 people who had donated a kidney between June 1, 1963 and December 31, 1979, with follow-up between 20–30 years. Of the donors, 84 had died and 380 were still alive. Three of the 84 donors who had died were known to have had kidney failure. Of the 380 donors who were still alive, three had abnormal kidney function and two had undergone transplantation. The remaining donors had normal kidney function. The rate of proteinuria and hypertension was similar to the age-matched general population. The risk of combined kidney failure in this study was 0.013% [36].

Limited initial evaluation

On initial evaluation of the recipient, a thorough family medical and psychosocial history may identify potential donors. Willing potential donors are then scheduled for an initial evaluation. Recipients with a strong familial history of diabetes or hypertension, certain glomerular diseases, or hereditary renal diseases should be cautioned about pursuing living donation from first-degree relatives, with preference given to second-degree relatives (cousins, nieces, nephews, uncles, or aunts) or unrelated persons. Donors from families with hereditary kidney diseases, such as autosomal dominant polycystic kidney disease and hereditary nephritis (eg, Alport's syndrome), who are >30 years old, with one or no cysts, or abnormalities of urinalysis may still be considered for donation.

Once potential candidates are identified, ABO blood-typing is performed and ABO-compatible donors are crossmatched and tissue-typed (human leukocyte antigen [HLA]-typing). Because the latter is an expensive procedure, some centers will defer tissue-typing until medical evaluation of the potential donor is complete. When multiple donors are evaluated at the same time, it is perhaps most cost-effective to perform tissue-typing and crossmatching first, in order to determine which individual is the optimal donor. An ABO-compatible donor who is crossmatch-negative and has the fewest HLA mismatches with the recipient is then scheduled for an expanded evaluation.

Expanded evaluation

The final evaluation of the donor requires a multidisciplinary approach (surgical team, nephrologist, transplant co-ordinators, internists, psychiatrists, social workers, and cardiologists). In order to reduce bias, however, the final decision on suitability should be made by physicians other than the surgical team [37–39].

Transplant co-ordinators play a major role in planning the sequence of tests listed in **Table 4**. Psychosocial evaluation should be performed to ensure that the donation is being offered voluntarily and with informed consent. Medical evaluation should be scheduled once routine tests and renal evaluation (24-hour urine for protein and creatinine, routine urinalysis, and ultrasonography of the kidneys) are completed. During evaluation, a complete personal and family history is obtained, and all laboratory tests are reviewed and discussed with the donor. In some transplant centers, the referring nephrologist will perform the donor medical evaluation. While convenient, one must caution that bias toward donation may be introduced if the nephrologist is also caring for the recipient.

Expanded living kidney donor evaluation
• Medical history and physical examinations, including multiple blood pressure determinations
• Psychosocial evaluation
• Routine tests: electrocardiogram, chest x-ray, complete blood count, blood chemistries for metabolic, renal, and hepatic function, lipid profile (for women: pregnancy test, Pap smear, mammogram for women >40 years)
• Screening for infection: CMV, EBV, HBsAg, HCV antibody, HIV
• Renal assessment: urinalysis, 24-hour urine for protein and creatinine, radionuclide GFR determination
• When indicated (see text): glycohemoglobin or oral glucose tolerance tests, ambulatory blood pressure monitoring, pulmonary function tests, noninvasive cardiac screening tests, lupus serologies, hemoglobin electrophoresis
• Tissue-typing and crossmatch
• Renal arteriogram, MRA, or spiral CT

Table 4. Expanded evaluation of living kidney donors. CMV: cytomegalovirus; CT: computed tomography; EBV: Epstein–Barr virus; GFR: glomerular filtration rate; HBsAg: hepatitis B surface antigen; HCV: hepatitis C virus; HIV: human immunodeficiency virus; MRA: magnetic resonance angiography; Pap: Papanicolaou.

In addition to medical suitability as a donor, appropriateness as a surgical candidate must also be assessed. When more than one donor is suitable, the older donor with best match should be selected so that the younger candidates can be preserved for future donation. There is no evidence that women who become pregnant following kidney donation are at increased risk for obstetric problems. However, if the recipient has hereditary renal disease, donors who have not yet started a family, or those with small children, must be reminded that, should one of their children later require transplantation, they would be unable to donate their remaining kidney.

In certain circumstances, additional testing may be required. In patients with isolated blood pressure readings in the hypertensive range, ambulatory blood pressure monitoring is helpful to determine whether the potential donor has "white coat" hypertension. For patients with a strong family history of diabetes, an oral glucose tolerance test or determination of glycosylated hemoglobin levels should be considered; anti-islet antibodies may be examined in first-degree relatives of patients with type 1 diabetes. At our center, a 24-hour urine protein of >150 mg requires repeat measurement for 8–12 hours in the supine position to rule out orthostatic proteinuria. Elevated 24-hour urine protein may sometimes result from excessive exercise during the collection period, and potential donors should be advised of this.

Pulmonary function tests may be necessary for long-term smokers, especially those with pulmonary symptoms, and noninvasive cardiac work-up may be recommended for patients with an abnormal electrocardiogram or multiple risk factors (such as hyperlipidemia and older age).

A renal biopsy may be required in donors with a family history of hereditary nephritis, especially in the presence of hematuria. Although most centers reject such donors, some will accept them if both biopsy and urologic examination are normal. Donors from families with adult polycystic kidney disease should have no more than two unilateral cysts, or one cyst in either kidney, before the age of 30 years. In one study, these criteria yielded a 99.2% positive predictive value and 100% negative predictive value for the presence of polycystic kidney disease, using PKD1 (polycystic kidney disease 1) DNA as the gold standard [40].

Donors with a family history of systemic lupus erythematosus should receive basic screening, including antinuclear antibody and serum complement levels. Following medical and surgical clearance, renal imaging by magnetic resonance or standard angiography is scheduled, and a date for donation arranged.

Contraindications to living kidney donation

Absolute contraindications for living kidney donation refer to those conditions that place the donor at high risk for kidney disease, or the recipient at high risk for development of neoplastic or infectious disease (see **Table 5**). Contraindications include extremes of age (<18 or >70 years old), ABO incompatibility, positive T-cell cytotoxic crossmatch, hypertension (as defined by blood pressure >140/90 mm Hg with or without medication), diabetes mellitus, HIV infection, hepatitis B or C infection, proteinuria, microscopic hematuria, creatinine clearance <60 mL/min, systemic disease with a potential for kidney involvement (such as lupus), malignancy, and active infection. While 24-hour protein >300 mg is generally rejected and <150 mg accepted for donation, there is center-wide variation in acceptance of protein values between 150–300 mg [37]. Microalbumin values >30 mg/day in donors with 24-hour protein excretion between 150–300 mg will identify those at risk for glomerular disease and therefore contraindicate donation. Abnormalities of the genitourinary tract, such as the presence of two or more renal cysts before the age of 30 years, recurrent nephrolithiasis, or abnormalities of the renal parenchyma or collecting system, are also contraindications for living donation.

Relative contraindications include incompatibility of the B-cell lymphocytotoxic or flow cytometric crossmatch, alcohol abuse with abstinence documented by history or a chemical-dependency program, drug abuse documented by abstinence (preferably by a chemical-dependency program), history of nephrolithiasis with no stones found on current renal imaging studies or abnormal urinary calcium excretion, moderate obesity (BMI >30 kg/m^2), hyperlipidemia, smoking, age >65 years (depending on the donor's "biological age"), family history of cardiovascular disease, and multiple cardiovascular risk factors without end organ damage.

Smaller programs often have more rigid criteria for donor selection, while bigger programs are more liberal in their

Contraindications to living kidney donation
• ABO incompatibility
• Positive T-cell cytotoxic crossmatch
• Age <18 or >70 years
• Newly diagnosed hypertension
• Hypertension, treated or not
• Diabetes
• Active chronic infection, such as HIV or hepatitis B
• Abnormal glucose tolerance test or glycohemoglobin
• Microalbuminuria or overt proteinuria
• Persistent microscopic hematuria on repeat urinalysis
• Strong family history of renal disease, type 2 diabetes, or hypertension
• GFR <80 mL/min (or <60 mL/min in some programs)
• Recurrent kidney stones
• Major anatomic disorder of donor kidneys
• Nephrolithiasis
• Medical contraindication to surgery, such as cardiopulmonary disease or malignancy, or other systemic disease
• History of thromboembolic disease
• Body mass index >30 kg/m^2
• Psychiatric contraindications or impaired decision-making capacity

Table 5. Contraindications to living kidney donation. GFR: glomerular filtration rate; HIV: human immunodeficiency virus.

approach: in a survey of US transplant centers, 59% had a cut-off of 80 mL/min for creatinine clearance, while 21% had a cut-off of 60 mL/min; the lower cut-off value was more likely to be found at the larger centers [41].

Ethical considerations of living kidney donation

The ethical considerations of living kidney donation are complex. Issues regarding coercion or financial gain must always be considered when evaluating a living donor. At some centers, an ethics committee is consulted for difficult cases, especially where there is no relationship between the donor and recipient, or where the relationship appears tenuous.

Even with related donation, it must be determined whether any emotional coercion has taken place (eg, via a "family meeting" or induction of guilt). Sometimes, assuring the potential donor in private that a "medical reason" for contraindication to transplantation can be found will elicit feelings of ambivalence or actual hostility toward the donation situation. Physicians have a responsibility to protect the well-being of both participants.

Conclusion

Kidney transplantation offers a chance of improved rehabilitation and quality of life for patients with end-stage renal disease. The choice of donor and recipient has a long-term impact on the course of the transplant itself. A patient in optimal medical condition prior to transplantation has the greatest potential for long-term survival in an era in which death with a functioning allograft has become a leading cause of graft loss. In a well-chosen living donor, there should be minimal medical impact on the donor's life from the procedure itself, and maximal emotional impact from the knowledge that his or her gift has given the recipient a new chance at life.

References

1. Massy ZA, Guijarro C, Wiederkehr MR et al. Chronic renal allograft rejection: immunologic and nonimmunologic risk factors. *Kidney Int* 1996;49:518–24.
2. Kasiske BL, Cangro CB, Hariharan S et al. American Society of Transplantation. The evaluation of renal transplantation candidates: clinical practice guidelines. *Am J Transplant* 2002;1(Suppl. 2):1–95.
3. Buhler LH, Spitzer TR, Sykes M et al. Induction of kidney allograft tolerance after transient lymphohematopietic chimerism in patients with multiple myeloma and end-stage renal disease. *Transplantation* 2002;74:1405-9.

4. Marcus R, Favero MS, Banerjee S et al. Prevalence and incidence of human immunodeficiency virus among patients undergoing long-term hemodialysis. The Cooperative Dialysis Study Group. *Am J Med* 1991;90:614–9.
5. Lago M, Perez-Garcia R, Garcia de Vinuesa MS et al. Human immunodeficiency virus infection in patients on maintenance dialysis. *Nephron* 1996;72:727 .
6. Spital A. Should all human immunodeficiency virus-infected patients with end-stage renal disease be excluded from transplantation? The views of U.S. transplant centers. *Transplantation* 1998;65:1187–91.
7. Swanson SJ, Kirk AD, Ko CW et al. Impact of HIV seropositivity on graft and patient survival after cadaveric renal transplantation in the United States in the pre highly active antiretroviral therapy (HAART) era: an historical cohort analysis of the United States Renal Data System. *Transpl Infect Dis* 2002;4:144–7.
8. Kuo PC, Stock PG. Transplantation in the HIV+ patient. *Am J Transplant* 2001;1:13–7.
9. Lloveras J, Peterson PK, Simmons RL et al. Mycobacterial infections in renal transplant recipients. Seven cases and a review of the literature. *Arch Intern Med* 1982;142:888–92.
10. Biz E, Pereira CA, Moura LA et al. The use of cyclosporine modifies the clinical and histopathological presentation of tuberculosis after renal transplantation. *Rev Inst Med Trop Sao Paulo* 2000;42:225–30.
11. Woeltje KF, Mathew A, Rothstein M et al. Tuberculosis infection and anergy in hemodialysis patients. *Am J Kidney Dis* 1998;31:848–52.
12. Sakhuja V, Jha V, Varma PP et al. The high incidence of tuberculosis among renal transplant recipients in India. *Transplantation* 1996;61:211–5 .
13. Bakir N, Surachno S, Sluiter WJ et al. Peritonitis in peritoneal dialysis patients after renal transplantation. *Nephrol Dial Transplant* 1998;13:3178–83.
14. Passalacqua JA, Wiland AM, Fink JC et al. Increased incidence of postoperative infections associated with peritoneal dialysis in renal transplant recipients. *Transplantation* 1999;68:535–40.
15. Leichter HE, Salusky IB, Ettenger RB et al. Experience with renal transplantation in children undergoing peritoneal dialysis (CAPD/CCPD). *Am J Kidney Dis* 1986;8:181–5.
16. Rangel MC, Coronado VG, Euler GL et al. Vaccine recommendations for patients on chronic dialysis. The Advisory Committee on Immunization Practices and the American Academy of Pediatrics. *Semin Dial* 2000;13:101–7.
17. Breitenfeldt MK, Rasenack J, Berthold H et al. Impact of hepatitis B and C on graft loss and mortality of patients after kidney transplantation. *Clin Transplant* 2002;16:130–6.
18. Kletzmayr J, Watschinger B. Chronic hepatitis B virus infection in renal transplant recipients. *Semin Nephrol* 2002;22:375–89.
19. Gane E, Pilmore H. Management of chronic viral hepatitis before and after renal transplantation. *Transplantation* 2002;74:427–37.
20. Jassal SV, Roscoe JM, Zaltzman JS et al. Clinical practice guidelines: prevention of cytomegalovirus disease after renal transplantation. *J Am Soc Nephrol* 1998;9:1697–708.
21. Sagedal S, Nordal KP, Hartmann A et al. A prospective study of the natural course of cytomegalovirus infection and disease in renal allograft recipients. *Transplantation* 2000;70:1166–74.
22. Beck J, Garcia R, Heiss G et al. Periodontal disease and cardiovascular disease. *J Periodontol* 1996;67(10 Suppl.):1123–37.
23. Lewis MS, Wilson RA, Walker K et al. Factors in cardiac risk stratification of candidates for renal transplant. *J Cardiovasc Risk* 1999;6:251–5.
24. Heston TF, Norman DJ, Barry JM et al. Cardiac risk stratification in renal transplantation using a form of artificial intelligence. *Am J Cardiol* 1997;79:415–7.
25. Cerilli J, Evans WE, Vaccaro PS. Successful simultaneous renal transplantation and abdominal aortic aneurysmectomy. *Arch Surg* 1977;112:1218–9.

26. Piquet P, Berland Y, Coulange C et al. Aortoiliac reconstruction and renal transplantation: staged or simultaneous. *Ann Vasc Surg* 1989;3:251–6.
27. Fritsche L, Vanrenterghem Y, Nordal KP et al. Practice variations in the evaluation of adult candidates for cadaveric kidney transplantation: a survey of the European Transplant Centers. *Transplantation* 2000;70:1492–7.
28. Danovitch GM, Hariharan S, Pirsch JD et al. Management of the waiting list for cadaveric kidney transplants: report of a survey and recommendations by the Clinical Practice Guidelines Committee of the American Society of Transplantation. *J Am Soc Nephrol* 2002;13:528–35.
29. Johnson DW, Isbel NM, Brown AM et al. The effect of obesity on renal transplant outcomes. *Transplantation* 2002;74:675–81.
30. Franco EL, Duarte-Franco E, Rohan TE. Evidence-based policy recommendations on cancer screening and prevention. *Cancer Detect Prev* 2002;26:350–61.
31. Kasiske BL, Snyder JJ, Matas AJ et al. Preemptive kidney transplantation: the advantage and the advantaged. *J Am Soc Nephrol* 2002;13:1358–64.
32. United Network for Organ Sharing (UNOS). Available from URL: http://www.unos.org
33. Wolfe RA, Ashby VB, Milford EL et al. Comparison of mortality in all patients on dialysis, patients on dialysis awaiting transplantation, and recipients of a first cadaveric transplant. *N Engl J Med* 1999;341:1725–30.
34. Bresnahan BA, McBride MA, Cherikh WS et al. Risk factors for renal allograft survival from pediatric cadaver donors: an analysis of United Network for Organ Sharing data. *Transplantation* 2001;72:256–61.
35. Gridelli B, Remuzzi G. Strategies for making more organs available for transplantation. *N Engl J Med* 2000;343:404–10.
36. Ramcharan T, Matas AJ. Long-term (20–37 years) follow-up of living kidney donors. *Am J Transplant* 2002;2:959–64.
37. Kasiske BL, Bia MJ. The evaluation and selection of living kidney donors. *Am J Kidney Dis* 1995;26:387–98.
38. Lumsdaine JA, Wigmore SJ, Forsythe JL. Live kidney donor assessment in the UK and Ireland. *Br J Surg* 1999;86:877–81
39. Kasiske BL, Ravenscraft M, Ramos EL et al. The evaluation of living renal transplant donors: clinical practice guidelines. Ad Hoc Clinical Practice Guidelines Subcommittee of the Patient Care and Education Committee of the American Society of Transplant Physicians. *J Am Soc Nephrol* 1996;7:2288–313.
40. Ravine D, Gibson RN, Walker RG et al. Evaluation of ultrasonographic diagnostic criteria for autosomal dominant polycystic kidney disease 1. *Lancet* 1994;343:824–7.
41. Bia MJ, Ramos EL, Danovitch GM et al. Evaluation of living renal donors. The current practice of US transplant centers. *Transplantation* 1995;60:322–7.

5

Surgical considerations in kidney transplantation

John F Valente & James A Schulak

Introduction

The field of kidney transplantation has grown tremendously since the first successful operation at the Peter Brent Brigham Hospital in Boston in 1954, where a live donor kidney was transplanted from one identical twin to his uremic brother. Currently, approximately 14,000 kidney transplants are performed in the US each year.

The techniques employed today to implant and revascularize a kidney transplant are essentially identical to those employed by Joseph E Murray and his colleagues in 1954 [1]. However, numerous innovations have been added to the surgical armamentarium of those who perform kidney transplantations, notably: implantation of *en bloc* pediatric kidneys; transplantation of two adult kidneys into one recipient; use of kidneys with vascular and anatomical anomalies; transplantation of kidneys simultaneously with the transplant of other abdominal organs; laparoscopic live donor nephrectomy; and the use of laparoscopic techniques and radiologically guided interventions to address postoperative complications.

This chapter reviews the surgical techniques that are employed to obtain kidneys from both living and deceased donors, perform kidney transplantation, and treat postoperative complications.

Donor selection and procurement

Cadaver donor selection

Cadaveric donors must meet criteria for death, either by pronouncement following withdrawal of life support (nonheart-beating donor) or by clinical criteria for brain death. In addition, legal consent must be given by the donor's family or personal designation (eg, driver's licence).

In general, donors with good renal function who range in age from birth to 70 years are acceptable. However, all donors >60 years old, and those >50 years with an elevated serum creatinine concentration, history of hypertension, or stroke as a cause of death, are categorized as "expanded criteria donors" [2]. This designation allows those recipients willing to accept organs from such donors to be separately listed and expeditiously matched for them. This strategy may reduce ischemia time and improve utilization of the aging donor pool.

The basic requirements for renal transplantation are HIV seronegativity, absence of active transmissible infection or malignancy, and sufficient hemodynamic stability to allow preservation (or at least recovery) of renal function. Patients with infections of the central nervous system (CNS) who are on appropriate antibiotic therapy, and those patients with primary CNS tumors in the absence of a ventriculo-peritoneal shunt or recent surgery, may be acceptable [3,4]. Prior abdominal surgery and the presence of intestinal stomas or feeding tubes are not contraindications to procurement.

Cadaver donor procurement

Heart-beating, kidney-only procurement

In cadaveric donors, anesthesia personnel provide monitoring support and maintain hemodynamic stability during the operative procedure. The following steps are involved:

- A midline incision is made from the xiphoid to the pubis

- The aorta is exposed at the iliac bifurcation for perfusion, and at the diaphragm for cross-clamping
- The left colon, right colon, and mesenteric root can be mobilized to give a wide exposure to the retroperitoneum
- The distal inferior vena cava is used for venting of venous effluent during perfusion
- Gerota's fascia is opened to allow ice packing closer to the kidneys
- After perfusion, the superior mesenteric artery (SMA) and porta-hepatis may be divided to further expose the suprarenal aorta

The kidneys are removed *en bloc* (ie, with the aorta and cava) and separated on a back table. Infant kidneys should be kept *en bloc* to facilitate combined transplantation. Because of its short length, the right renal vein is usually left attached to the entire vena cava. Perinephric fat should be cleared and superficial cysts opened to screen for carcinomas. Biopsy sites should be sutured closed. Horseshoe or other ectopic kidneys are usable if the vascular supply is suitable.

Heart-beating, multiorgan procurement

Multiorgan procurement follows an established sequence designed to maximize organ recovery, minimize loss of life-saving organs, and provide adequate exposure. A median sternotomy and laparotomy allow for isolation of the great vessels in the chest, diaphragm, and iliac bifurcation. This provides exposure for rapid cannulation in case of donor instability. Further dissection to document anatomic variations, assess organ quality, and prepare for extirpation is best kept to a minimum.

As with kidney-only procurement, organ removal is preceded by transaortic perfusion with cold preservation solution. Organ removal occurs in a standard order: heart, lung(s), liver, pancreas, and kidney. The procurement team must take care to avoid excess renal warm ischemia time while attention is focused on the liver and pancreas.

Nonheart-beating procurement

All procurement activities must follow the legal declaration of death. Periods of agonal respiration and low blood pressure add to warm ischemia, which may limit organ viability and preclude donation. When life support is withdrawn, close proximity to the operating room is preferred.

Rapid vascular cannulation and organ cooling is the first goal, and should be accomplished by prompt laparotomy or introduction of specialized arterial and venous catheters for cold perfusion. When the organs are cool, removal is performed as described above. Suitable kidney, liver, pancreas, and lung allografts have been obtained from nonheart-beating donors [5,6].

Organ preservation

Kidneys may be preserved for up to 72 hours, but use within <24 hours minimizes the risk of delayed graft function (DGF). University of Wisconsin (UW, Viaspan, Dupont) solution is commonly used for both perfusion and storage. Preservation solutions are high in oncotic pressure and are similar to intracellular electrolyte concentrations in order to prevent cellular swelling.

Simple cold storage is adequate for short periods, but for storage >24 hours, a pulsatile preservation pump should be used to optimize preservation. The latter is associated with a decrease in the incidence of graft dysfunction, and may be used to monitor trends in perfusion pressure and vascular resistance [7]. Ischemia-reperfusion injury is common, and numerous pharmacologic and biologic interventions that may minimize the incidence of subsequent DGF are being investigated.

Live donor selection

Healthy adults with an emotional attachment to the recipient are the usual candidates for kidney donation, but emotionally unattached donors and donor pools shared between families may also be considered. Requisites for donation include:

- ABO blood-group compatibility
- lack of chronic infection (especially with HIV or hepatitis)
- a malignancy-free state
- psychosocial stability
- informed consent
- an absence of conditions likely to cause impairment of renal function over time

The criteria for donor selection are discussed in detail in Chapter 4. Kidney selection is based on the principle of *primum non nocere*, ie, in cases of significant disparity, the kidney with best potential for long-term function must remain with the donor. Arterial and ureteral anatomy must be determined. This may be achieved with conventional angiography, spiral computed tomography with image reconstruction, or magnetic resonance imaging. The kidney with the simplest anatomy is preferred. The left kidney is usually chosen because it has a longer vein.

Live donor procurement

Open nephrectomy

Traditionally, open nephrectomy has been performed through a flank incision that sacrifices the tip of the 12th rib, and extends to the border of the rectus muscle. Smaller, less painful incisions are now preferred, and provide postoperative recovery times similar to laparoscopic methods [8].

The vascular supply is exposed for an adequate length. The adrenal is spared and the ureter cleared for 10–15 cm. After systemic anticoagulation, both artery and vein are transected under the control of vascular clamps. Vessel stumps are secured with suture or staples. Care must be taken to prevent dislodgement of the clamp in order to decrease the risk of significant blood loss. During closure, intercostal nerve entrapment is a complication that can lead to chronic pain and disability.

Patients are discharged in 3–5 days, and postoperative convalescence usually requires 4–6 weeks.

Laparoscopic nephrectomy

Laparoscopic donor nephrectomy, first reported in 1995, was initially reserved for left kidneys with standard anatomy, and was associated with a slightly increased risk for DGF compared with open donors [9]. Currently, with increased use of the hand-assisted approach, right kidneys and grafts with multiple renal arteries are frequently obtained, all with good results [10]. Previous extensive abdominal surgery that involved the retroperitoneal/perinephric tissue planes is a major contraindication to laparoscopic donation.

Safety dictates starting with a blunt cannula or initial placement of the hand port. The latter requires a lateral, muscle-splitting incision or a small midline fascial incision. During dissection, inflation pressures are kept below 10–12 mm Hg, and intravenous fluids are administered generously to minimize renal dysfunction.

The transperitoneal approach involves mobilization of the colon and duodenum (for the right kidney). Once dissection is complete, a brief period of deflation helps to establish a brisk diuresis. The vessels are secured using an endo-"thoracic/abdominal" stapler or an endovascular "gastrointestinal anastomosis" stapler. For shorter vessels, the single-row stapler followed by transection with scissors affords greater length. The kidney is removed through the hand-port.

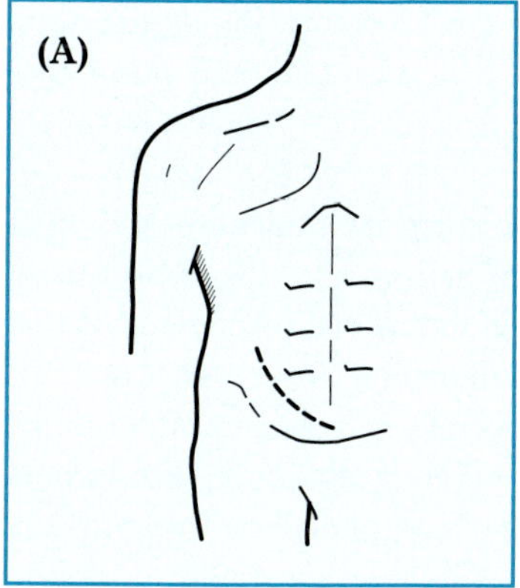

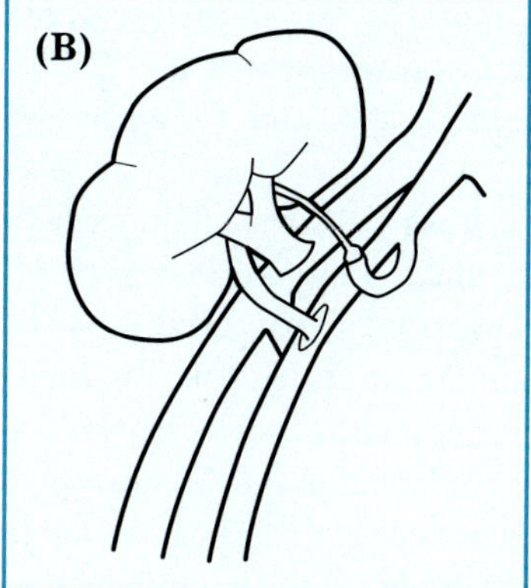

Figure 1. (**A**) The standard lower quadrant incision allows access to the retroperitoneum. (**B**) The final anatomy of a revascularized renal allograft. Note the use of the internal iliac artery as a separate inflow for the polar renal artery.

Preoperative counseling about initial postoperative discomfort and attention to early pain control help to foster postoperative independence and early discharge.

Recipient transplantation

Adult transplantation

Single kidney implantation

The extraperitoneal approach, using the iliac vessels for blood supply, has been the mainstay for single kidney transplantation since its inception (see **Figure 1**). In most cases, preoperative physical examination and review of previously obtained noninvasive testing are sufficient to ensure an adequate arterial supply. Patients with long waiting times and disease progression require a careful approach to preoperative clearance, even if this is limited to the day of cadaveric transplantation.

Care is required when severely atherosclerotic vessels are encountered in order to prevent injury to the leg or compromised renal blood flow. The recipient's saphenous vein can be used as a conduit to extend the renal artery if it is too short. Rarely, excision and replacement of the iliac artery with a prosthetic conduit can provide a location for anastomosis.

Aorto-iliac disease that precludes safe arterial implantation should be diagnosed and bypassed prior to listing, allowing subsequent transplant to the bypass graft. Intra-abdominal placement of the kidney to utilize the proximal common iliac vessels or even the aorta is occasionally necessary, especially in patients undergoing retransplantation. Venous length is rarely an issue, but, when necessary, very short veins can be lengthened by creating an extension graft using the donor vena cava or a segment of donor iliac vein.

The technique for ureteral implantation depends upon the anatomy of the patient and the preference of the surgeon. The anterior (Gregoir–Lich) ureteroneocystostomy is straightforward and most common, but slightly more prone to leak than the posterior (Ledbetter) approach. A uretero (recipient)–pyelostomy (donor) or direct ureter-to-ureter anastomosis can be used when the donor ureter is short or the bladder is small. If necessary, ureteral implantation to an augmented bladder, ileal conduit, or even construction of a cutaneous ureterostomy can be performed.

In general, construction of an ileal loop or bladder augmentation should be performed prior to transplantation in order to decrease the incidence of postoperative complications.

Dual adult kidney implantation

When the donor biopsy shows significant glomerulosclerosis (>25%) and the anticipated creatinine clearance from a single kidney is low (<30–40 mL/min), the implantation of both kidneys from a cadaveric donor into a single recipient is a viable strategy [11].

Both grafts are generally placed on the same side to avoid the morbidity of bilateral incisions. The first allograft is placed

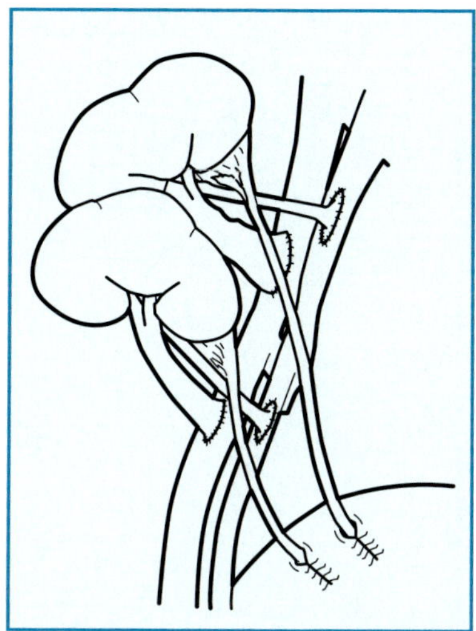

Figure 2. The positioning of "two for one" kidneys from donors with low creatinine clearance can be performed down one side, avoiding the more extensive bilateral approach. In such cases, implantation of the right kidney is facilitated by creating a venous extension, utilizing the vena cava. This technique leaves the contralateral iliac vessels unaltered, facilitating future retransplantation.

relatively high on the external or common iliac vessels. The vascular clamps are then moved below the first kidney, allowing it to perfuse, while the second kidney is implanted distally on the external iliac vessels (see **Figure 2**). Alternatively, the kidneys can be placed bilaterally through a single midline incision.

Results of "two for one" transplants are comparable with, or even exceed, those from single, ideal kidneys [12]. Unfortunately, patients with extensive atherosclerosis are relatively poor candidates for this approach.

En bloc pediatric kidney implantation

In most situations, pediatric kidneys used individually are quite acceptable for adult recipients, as the grafts hypertrophy and ultimately function well. However, kidneys from donors weighing <20 kg have diminutive renal vasculature, which increases the risk

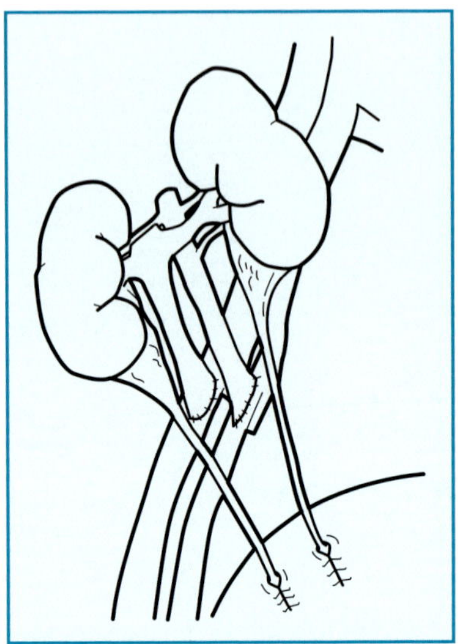

Figure 3. Pediatric kidneys, when used *en bloc*, can be positioned on one side of the pelvis. The aorta and vena cava are used as conduits for revascularization. The ureters are implanted independently. Care must be taken to avoid vessel kinking when positioning the two kidneys prior to closure.

of technical failure, and may not provide adequate nephron mass for large adult recipients. Such kidneys may be kept *en bloc*, using the donor aorta and cava for anastomosis (see **Figure 3**).

Allograft survival is excellent when using pediatric kidneys *en bloc* from donors >1 year of age [13]. Special care must be taken to avoid vascular torsion, as the peritoneal contents are allowed to compress the kidneys laterally. Suture pexy of the grafts into a position promoting good blood flow, as assessed by intraoperative Doppler interrogation of each graft independently, is helpful. Mounting the kidneys on a sheet of absorbable mesh can be attempted if torsion seems unavoidable [14].

Kidney retransplantation

While a second transplant is easily accomplished by placement of the graft on the contralateral side, third and further retransplants require that the procedure take place in a reoperative field. Immunosuppression, prior infection, fluid collection, and occurrence of other surgical complications make the degree of scarring unpredictable. The procedure may require transplant nephrectomy and/or use of the iliac vessels higher than the previous anastomosis. Occasionally, an intraperitoneal approach with vascular reconstruction using the aorta and vena cava may be necessary.

Kidney transplantation in combination with other abdominal organs

Combined transplantation with the pancreas is routine, and is usually performed through a midline, intraperitoneal approach. Most surgeons prefer to transplant the kidney to the left side and the pancreas to the right, using the iliac vessels for both. Portal venous drainage for the pancreas moves the graft to the mid abdomen, away from the pelvis, affording greater options for kidney placement.

For patients with irreversible renal failure who are undergoing liver transplantation, a combined kidney–liver transplant is performed sequentially, through separate incisions. When the recipient is highly sensitized, transplantation of the liver first may allow for adsorption of preformed antibodies, thereby reducing the potential crossmatch barrier to kidney transplantation. If significant difficulties arise during liver implantation, the patient is stabilized in the intensive care unit and returned to the operating room for renal implantation in 12–18 hours.

Pediatric transplantation

Children accrue the greatest potential benefit from renal transplantation, but will also be exposed to the longest period of immunosuppression and have the longest requirement for good graft function. Consequently, ideal donor kidneys should be accepted for children (and perhaps young adults) unless urgent transplantation is required for some reason, such as impending loss of dialysis access [15].

Small vessel size, whether in the recipient or donor, increases the risk of vascular thrombosis when compared with adults. Moreover, the use of a pediatric donor for a pediatric recipient may compound this risk. Nevertheless, meticulous attention to surgical technique can result in excellent pediatric donor to pediatric recipient outcomes.

The standard, extraperitoneal approach is possible in most cases, but intra-abdominal transplantation using the aorta and vena cava is often the preferred technique for infants and children weighing <20 kg. Again, bladder reconstruction prior to or following transplantation should be weighed against the risks of urinary diversion at the time of transplant [16].

Surgical complications

Lymphocele, hematoma, and infection

Fluid collections following transplantation are common and consist of seromas, hematomas, and lymph collections. Lymphatics that drain the lower extremities surround the iliac vessels, and some are routinely divided at the time of transplantation, as are those in the hilum of the kidney allograft. Suture ligation of these channels is routine, but leakage of lymph occurs in 5%–15% of patients. Incidental collections that do not cause symptoms or renal dysfunction do not require intervention.

Lymphoceles that partially occlude the ureter or renal vein lead to renal dysfunction, and those compressing the iliac vein may cause ipsilateral leg swelling. Anatomic verification is obtained by either ultrasound or computerized tomography. Percutaneous drainage can be used to confirm the presence of lymphocytes in the fluid and establish the absence of infection, but simple drainage may be ineffective if the leak persists.

The most definitive approach involves unroofing of the lymphocele into the peritoneal cavity, allowing the lymphatic fluid to be reabsorbed in the peritoneum. This can be accomplished either laparoscopically or by a traditional open laparotomy. In either case, care must be taken to avoid injury to either the renal vessels or ureter [17].

Significant postoperative hemorrhage should be addressed by re-exploration. Large, stable hematomas may cause pain, become infected, or cause compression symptoms similar to lymphoceles, and should be evacuated. Wound infection above the level of the fascia is addressed with the same methods used in nontransplant surgery: open drainage, antibiotics, and local wound care. Deep-space infections must be adequately drained and aggressively controlled to avoid breakdown of vascular anastomoses.

While mycotic aneurysm formation is rare following renal transplantation, the condition will lead to hemorrhage and carries a high mortality rate (>50%) if not repaired expeditiously. Saphenous vein bypass to hilar arteries can be used to salvage the kidney. Allograft salvage may not be possible, however, when treating severe vascular infections and is of secondary consideration under these circumstances. Complete excision of the arterial anastomosis and vein patch repair are mandatory.

Urologic complications

Early urine leak and late ureteral stenosis are both rare, but important, complications following renal transplantation. Leaks occur in 1%–3% of cases, but may be more common when wound healing is impaired. Leakage from the anastomosis within days of transplantation is the most common scenario.

With small leaks, prolonged bladder drainage and ureteral stenting may lead to spontaneous healing, but repair is often necessary [18]. When feasible, repeat implantation into the bladder is the preferred technique, but a ureteroureterostomy or bladder flap is often required. Ureter implantation into a very small, spastic bladder can lead to calyceal blow-out, which results in a high-output leak from the kidney itself.

Transcutaneous stenting and prolonged drainage may lead to closure in some cases; however, surgical repair and bladder augmentation are often required to provide a low-pressure system with adequate capacitance. Stenosis may be due to ischemia, technical problems, or vascular rejection; hydronephrosis is the usual consequence. Either percutaneous, antegrade contrast study or transcytoscopic ureterography may be used to identify the stenotic area. Focal stenoses may be transluminally dilated and stented. Longer segments or recurrent stenoses usually require surgical reconstruction.

Elderly men may experience urinary retention following transplantation. This is kept to a minimum with appropriate preoperative screening, and a period of catheter drainage and pharmacologic therapy leads to resolution.

Vascular complications

The most common vascular complications following kidney transplantation include bleeding, thrombosis, pseudoaneurysm due to infection, and late arterial stenosis. Arterial thrombosis occurs in 1%–2% of patients [19], and may arise from technical errors, hypercoagulability [20], increased vascular resistance in the allograft, or occlusion/thrombosis of the native vessel used for reconstruction. Immediate recognition is necessary if salvage is to be achieved.

In patients previously exhibiting a diuresis, sudden anuria is highly suggestive of thrombosis, but, in the setting of DGF, early arterial occlusion must be detected by imaging techniques such as Doppler ultrasonography. Arterial thrombosis requires an urgent return to the operating room for confirmation, thrombectomy, infusion of thrombolytic agents, and correction of any technical errors. In most cases, renal function will not be restored, and transplant nephrectomy will be necessary.

Isolated venous thrombosis can cause hematuria and allograft dysfunction and, like arterial thrombosis, is rarely reversible.

Late renal artery stenosis may present with hypertension, allograft dysfunction, or both. Conventional or carbon dioxide angiography or magnetic resonance imaging may yield the diagnosis. Short-segment stenoses may be amenable to angiographic dilation and stenting. Long-segment arterial narrowing or a tortuous artery may preclude angioplasty, making renal/artery bypass the only option. A renal artery bypass with the saphenous vein is useful in such situations, if residual graft function is anticipated to merit the procedure.

Parenchymal injury

Acute swelling/congestion of an allograft, either from venous occlusion, severe acute rejection, or both, can lead to parenchymal fractures and hemorrhage [21]. In some cases, reoperation to control bleeding, address outflow issues by thrombectomy, and correct venous kinks may lead to allograft salvage.

Transplant nephrectomy

Indications

Absolute indications for transplant nephrectomy include: hyperacute rejection, unremitting hemorrhage (wound or urinary tract), early arterial or venous thrombosis, mycotic aneurysm formation at the vascular anastomosis, or systemic illness and thrombocytopenia with DGF due to drug-induced hemolytic-uremic syndrome or severe rejection.

Indications for selective transplant nephrectomy include: persistent DGF lasting >8 weeks without signs of improvement, chronic infection or severe pain in a nonfunctioning kidney, severe proteinuria or systemic complications refractory to medical management, and renal artery-related hypertension that is not amenable to angioinvasive or operative intervention.

Relative indications for transplant nephrectomy include: early graft failure (<3 months) in live donor recipients with additional living-related donors, graft failure at any time in a highly sensitized patient (pretransplant panel-reactive antibodies >50%), and patient preference.

Nephrectomy may also be indicated for pain and swelling following withdrawal of immunosuppression in failed transplants. Tumors, often due to lymphoproliferative disorders, are less common indications for allograft nephrectomy, but, when present, necessitate the procedure.

Surgical technique

Early transplant nephrectomy is a rapid, simple procedure. In most cases, division of the vessels is simplified if a donor vascular patch is left in place. Otherwise, a vein patch repair of the iliac artery is required. Complete excision of the ureter and reclosure of the bladder is easy and is usually performed.

Late nephrectomy following scar formation is best accomplished through a limited incision directly over the allograft. The renal capsule is entered and the kidney easily shelled out, exposing the hilum. Intracapsular dissection avoids injury to the iliac vessels and other recipient structures. Significant hemorrhage is occasionally encountered, and expeditious cross-clamping at the hilum allows for rapid excision of the kidney. Vessels are individually sutured.

While it is not necessary to completely remove the ureter unless a specific indication exists, the renal pelvis should be excised to prevent development of a vascular-vesical fistula.

Complications

Apart from the routine problems common to all operations, transplant nephrectomy involves the particular risks of vascular and nerve injury owing to the scarred reoperative field. Limited use of mechanical retraction and avoidance of unnecessary dissection are important rules.

Persistent hematuria following nephrectomy may rarely be due to an arterial–ureteral fistula (see above), but is usually indicative of an inadequate preoperative work-up and misdiagnosis of the transplant as the cause of bladder hemorrhage.

Postoperative infection risks are greater when pyelonephritis is the indication for nephrectomy. Perioperative antibiotics must be based on culture-proven sensitivities. Brief reliance on closed suction helps to reduce fluid collections, and the drain can be removed within 48 hours of the procedure.

Conclusion

The approach to single kidney renal transplantation has not changed in any substantial way for several decades, but broader patient acceptance and utilization of wider donor criteria have brought a number of technical challenges to the field. Over the last decade, laparoscopic donation represents the single greatest technical change in the live donor process.

Surgical complications and risks are well defined for transplantation and its associated procedures. The incidence of adverse events depends upon medication effects, graft function, and donor/recipient factors. The impact of modern immunosuppressive agents on healing and postoperative surgical complications is likely to be felt more sharply in the future, as new and more powerful agents are introduced.

References

1. Merrill JP, Murray JE, Harrison JH et al. Successful homotransplantation of the human kidney between identical twins. *JAMA* 1956;160:277–82.
2. Basar H, Soran A, Shapiro R et al. Renal transplantation in recipients over the age of 60: the impact of donor age. *Transplantation* 1999;67:1191–3.
3. Kauffman HM, McBride MA, Cherikh WS et al. Transplant tumor registry: donors with central nervous system tumors. *Transplantation* 2002;73:579–82.
4. Fecteau AH, Penn I, Hanto DW. Peritoneal metastasis of intracranial glioblastoma via a ventriculoperitoneal shunt preventing organ retrieval: case report and review of the literature. *Clin Transplant* 1998;12:348–50.

5. Balupuri S, Buckley P, Snowden C et al. The trouble with kidneys derived from the non heart-beating donor: a single center 10-year experience. *Transplantation* 2000;69:842–6.
6. D'Alessandro AM, Odorico JS, Knechtle SJ et al. Simultaneous pancreas–kidney (SPK) transplantation from controlled non-heart-beating donors (NHBDs). *Cell Transplant* 2000;9:889–93.
7. Polyak MM, Arrington BO, Stubenbord WT et al. The influence of pulsatile preservation on renal transplantation in the 1990s. *Transplantation* 2000;69:249–58.
8. Redman JF. An anterior extraperitoneal incision for donor nephrectomy that spares the rectus abdominis muscle and anterior abdominal wall nerves. *J Urol* 2000; 164:1898–900.
9. Ratner LE, Ciseck LJ, Moore RG et al. Laparoscopic live donor nephrectomy. *Transplantation* 1995;60:1047–9.
10. Wolf JS Jr, Merion RM, Leichtman AB et al. Randomized controlled trial of hand-assisted laparoscopic versus open surgical live donor nephrectomy. *Transplantation* 2001;72:284–90.
11. Andres A, Morales JM, Herrero JC et al. Double versus single renal allografts from aged donors. *Transplantation* 2000;69:2060–6.
12. Dietl KH, Wolters H, Marschall B et al. Cadaveric "two-in-one" kidney transplantation from marginal donors: experience of 26 cases after 3 years. *Transplantation* 2000; 70:790–4.
13. Strey C, Grotz W, Mutz C et al. Graft survival and graft function of pediatric en bloc kidneys in paraaortal position. *Transplantation* 2002;73:1095–9.
14. Chinnakotla S, Leone JP, Taylor RJ. Long-term results of en bloc transplantation of pediatric kidneys into adults using a vicryl mesh envelope technique. *Clin Transplant* 2001;15:388–92.
15. Kumar MS, Panigrahi D, Dezii CM et al. Long-term function and survival of elderly donor kidneys transplanted into young adults. *Transplantation* 1998;65:282–5.
16. Koo HP, Bunchman TE, Flynn JT et al. Renal transplantation in children with severe lower urinary tract dysfunction. *J Urol* 1999;161:240–5.
17. Melvin WS, Bumgardner GL, Davies EA et al. The laparoscopic management of post-transplant lymphocele. A critical review. *Surg Endosc* 1997;11:245–8.
18. van Roijen JH, Kirkels WJ, Zietse R et al. Long-term graft survival after urological complications of 695 kidney transplantations. *J Urol* 2001;165:1884–7.
19. Bakir N, Sluiter WJ, Ploeg RJ et al. Primary renal graft thrombosis. *Nephrol Dial Transplant* 1996;11:140–7.
20. Friedman GS, Meier-Kriesche HU, Kaplan B et al. Hypercoagulable states in renal transplant candidates: impact of anticoagulation upon incidence of renal allograft thrombosis. *Transplantation* 2001;72:1073–8.
21. Hochleitner BW, Kafka R, Spechtenhauser B et al. Renal allograft rupture is associated with rejection or acute tubular necrosis, but not with renal vein thrombosis. *Nephrol Dial Transplant* 2001;16:124–7.

6

Long-term complications of kidney transplantation

John D Pirsch

Introduction

Over 200,000 kidney transplants have been performed in the US since the early 1960s, and it is estimated that 100,000 kidney transplant recipients are currently alive with a functioning graft [1]. One-year kidney graft survival increased from 84.9% in 1994 to 90.3% in 1999 [2]. Although this is only a small improvement, the graft half-life increased from 11.1 years to 18.2 years in the same time period. These improvements in patient and graft survival have resulted in a large number of transplanted recipients who are at risk for immunosuppression-related complications. Further improvements in patient survival will only occur with a reduction in the comorbidity associated with transplantation and long-term immunosuppression.

The long-term complications of kidney transplantation are the result of a complex interaction between the medical condition of the recipient at the time of transplantation, the quality of the donor organ, and side effects of chronic immunosuppression maintenance. Patients presenting with end-stage renal disease often have significant comorbidities, including coronary artery disease, hypertension, hyperlipidemia, and diabetes mellitus [3].

Kidneys transplanted from living donors survive longer than those from cadavers [1,4]. The increasing use of older cadaver donors (>50 years of age) during the past decade has also influenced long-term graft survival, since kidneys from older donors have a higher rate of graft failure [4,5]. Finally, the long-term impact of chronic immunosuppression on cardiovascular risk factors and the risk of malignancy contributes to premature patient death following transplantation.

Until recently, little emphasis has been placed on the amelioration of long-term risk factors for mortality in kidney transplant recipients. During the 1990s, a number of important studies demonstrated the benefits of reducing cardiovascular risk factors in the general population [6–10]. Although formal studies of risk factor reduction have not been carried out in transplant recipients, there is no *a priori* reason to think that risk reduction will not be beneficial in this population.

In addition, effective therapies for the prevention of posttransplant bone disease have been developed and are commonly used in posttransplant recipients [11–13]. Finally, improvements in long-term immunosuppression have allowed avoidance or sparing of corticosteroid or calcineurin inhibitor therapy in some patients, resulting in an overall reduction in long-term immunosuppression [14–16].

This chapter reviews the most common posttransplant problems, including management of the kidney allograft, hypertension, hyperlipidemia, ischemic heart disease (IHD), and metabolic bone disease.

Management of the long-term kidney allograft

The long-term survival of a kidney allograft is highly dependent on whether the kidney is from a living or cadaveric donor. From 1995 to 1999, the projected half-life of a living donor organ in the US was 17.7 years compared with 10.9 years for a cadaver donor organ [1]. Since 1995, very few transplanted kidneys have been lost in the first year: the most recent 1-year and 5-year kidney graft survival rates are shown in **Figure 1**.

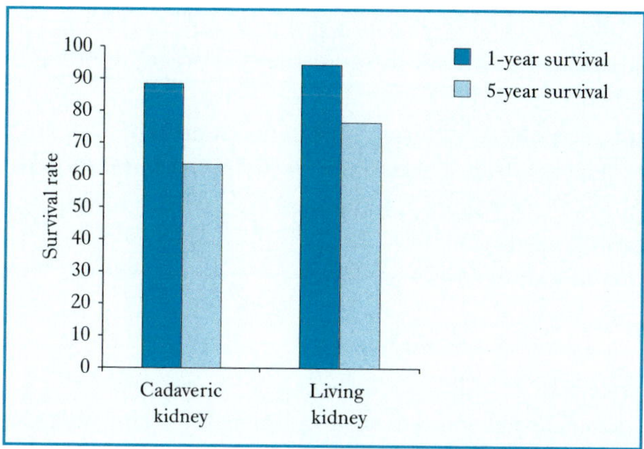

Figure 1. One-year graft survival rates reported for the 1999–2000 transplant recipient cohort; 5-year graft survival rates reported for the 1995–1996 cohort. The Organ Procurement and Transplantation Network data as of August 1, 2002.

During the first year posttransplant, patient death accounts for 25%–30% of all graft failures, and acute rejection for 20% [1]. After 1 year, chronic allograft nephropathy (CAN) is responsible for 27%–40% of graft failures, while patient death accounts for 35%–40%. Less than 10% of graft losses after 1 year are due to acute rejection, while infection, recurrent disease, and noncompliance account for the remainder. The main goal of long-term management is to maximize the longevity of the allograft and prevent premature mortality of the recipient.

Chronic allograft nephropathy

CAN is a slow deterioration of kidney function that may occur in long-term kidney transplant recipients [17,18]. On kidney biopsy, it is characterized by the presence of concentric intimal thickening of the small arterioles, interstitial fibrosis, tubular atrophy, and glomerulosclerosis [17]. The histologic changes are due to progressive ischemic injury from small blood vessel obliteration. The etiology of CAN is unknown, but it is clearly associated with both nonimmunologic and immunologic conditions.

Nonimmunologic associations include donor source (living or cadaver), cold-ischemia time of the transplanted organ, donor age and cause of death (eg, cerebrovascular accident vs. motor vehicle accident), and length of dialysis prior to transplant [19,20]. Immunologic factors that contribute to CAN include human leukocyte antigen mismatch, sensitization of the recipient, retransplantation, and rejection following transplant [21,22]. Alone or in combination, these factors may increase the risk for developing CAN.

Treatment of CAN

There is no generally accepted treatment for CAN. Many centers decrease or eliminate calcineurin inhibitors, since these drugs decrease renal blood flow through afferent arteriolar vasoconstriction [23–25]. Control of blood pressure with angiotensin-converting enzyme (ACE) inhibitors or angiotensin receptor blockers (ARBs) may slow the progression of CAN [26–28].

There is no convincing evidence that the addition of mycophenolate mofetil (MMF) or sirolimus can alter the progression of CAN. These drugs, however, may allow discontinuation of calcineurin inhibitors, a "conversion" strategy that is associated with a 5%–15% risk of inducing an acute rejection episode [29–31].

Chronic calcineurin inhibitor therapy

In the early 1980s, the introduction of the calcineurin inhibitor cyclosporine (CsA) revolutionized transplantation by improving short-term graft survival through a dramatic decrease in the severity and incidence of acute rejection episodes in the early posttransplant period. However, it immediately became apparent that CsA causes significant nephrotoxicity and renal failure in cardiac transplant recipients [32].

Concern over the use of calcineurin inhibitors (eg, CsA or tacrolimus) is well founded. Calcineurin inhibitors reduce renal blood flow by vasoconstriction of the afferent arteriole of the renal glomerulus [33]. The mechanism of action is unclear, but appears to involve release of endothelin-1 [34,35], decreased production of nitric oxide [36,37], and increased expression of transforming growth factor-β [38,39]. Chronic CsA toxicity is characterized by hyalinosis of the afferent arteriole with interstitial fibrosis, which is induced by chronic vasoconstriction.

Because of the potential for nephrotoxicity, various regimens have been employed in an effort to minimize the risk of calcineurin inhibitor therapy [40,41]. A number of groups have investigated calcineurin inhibitor withdrawal. Most transplant recipients can be successfully withdrawn from calcineurin inhibitors without rejection [4,40,42–45]. However, in some studies, up to 20% of patients developed acute rejection episodes.

In the early 1990s, data accumulated to suggest that, despite the impairment of renal function by CsA, most kidney transplants had stable function over at least a 5-year period [46]. There was also mounting evidence that acute rejection episodes, particularly late episodes, led to a higher risk of CAN [20,47,48].

At the present time, most kidney transplant recipients are managed with the lowest dose of CsA or tacrolimus possible. Target drug levels for chronic calcineurin inhibitor therapy are highly dependent on the risk of the individual recipient for acute rejection or graft failure. Thus, higher-risk recipients – such as younger patients (<30 years of age), African Americans, mismatched cadaver renal transplants, retransplant recipients, and recipients with previous acute rejection episodes – require higher levels of calcineurin immunosuppressants or additional immunosuppressant drugs (eg, MMF or sirolimus).

Posttransplant hypertension

In the posttransplant period, hypertension occurs in up to 80% of recipients [49]. In a recently completed 5-year cadaveric renal transplant trial, which compared tacrolimus with CsA, antihypertensive therapy was required in 81% of tacrolimus-treated and 90% of CsA-treated transplant recipients [49].

Hypertension in the recipient appears to be associated with poorer long-term graft survival. A large registry study showed that recipients with well-controlled blood pressure (<140 mm Hg systolic and <90 mm Hg diastolic) have improved long-term survival [50]. Although this relationship appears to be clear, this study was retrospective, and blood pressure control may actually be a surrogate marker for the quality of the donor organ. No prospective trials have yet assessed the level of blood pressure control in relation to long-term survival.

Posttransplant hypertension is a complex and multifactorial problem. Its underlying causes include renal insufficiency, calcineurin inhibitor and prednisone therapy, recurrent disease, renal artery stenosis (RAS) in the remnant native or transplant kidney, obesity, essential hypertension, and rejection [51–53]. In addition, transmission of hypertension from the donor to the recipient has been described [54].

Reduced blood flow to the kidney transplant activates the renin–angiotensin system, causing sodium retention, volume expansion, and hypertension. Impaired renal blood flow to the transplant may occur in a number of ways, including RAS, native iliac artery disease causing decreased kidney blood flow (pseudo-RAS), disease of the intraparenchymal renal arterioles from pre-existing donor vascular disease or CAN, or impaired cardiac output from pump failure. Conventional angiography is the gold standard for diagnosis. Ultrasound may be useful to screen for RAS, but is highly operator-dependent, with poor sensitivity and specificity. Recently, magnetic resonance angiography of the transplant has emerged as an effective modality for the detection of RAS and pseudo-RAS. This procedure is minimally invasive, and nephrotoxic contrast dye can be avoided [55].

A number of randomized controlled trials have studied the effects of blood pressure agents in kidney transplant recipients. Most of these have involved the use of calcium channel blockers (CCBs), since these drugs may improve afferent arteriolar flow into the glomerulus, and offset the effect of calcineurin inhibitors. The dihydropyridine CCBs are clearly effective in the management of posttransplant hypertension [56–58].

A randomized study comparing nifedipine (a CCB) and lisinopril (an ACE inhibitor) demonstrated improved renal outcomes (lower creatinine and improved glomerular filtration rate at 2 years) with nifedipine, but not lisinopril [57]. ACE inhibitors may cause minor deterioration of renal function, but also cause anemia in kidney transplant recipients receiving CsA or tacrolimus, which may explain the reluctance of transplant physicians to use these agents as an initial therapy for posttransplant hypertension.

Beta-blockers are also effective in the management of posttransplant hypertension. Because most transplant recipients are at risk for, or have, IHD, beta-blockers should be considered for adjunctive therapy. Other blood pressure-lowering agents, such as diuretics and alpha-blockers, are useful in recipients who require multiple medications for blood pressure control. The available agents are described in **Table 1**.

Hyperlipidemia

Hyperlipidemia affects 60%–80% of long-term kidney transplant recipients [59]. Associated risk factors for hyperlipidemia include poor kidney function, pretransplant hyperlipidemia, proteinuria, diabetes, some antihypertensive therapies (eg, nonselective beta-blockers and diuretics), and immunosuppression. Posttransplant

Class	Advantages	Disadvantages and side effects
Diuretics (furosemide, bumetanide, torsemide)	Useful for sodium retention and edema	Volume contraction, K^+, Mg^+ wasting, increased uric acid
Adrenergic inhibitors (clonidine, doxazosin, terazosin)	Clonidine is useful in diabetes, alpha-blockers in urinary retention	Postural hypotension, sedation
Beta-blockers (atenolol, labetalol, metoprolol)	Useful in recipients with IHD and in combination therapy with CCB	Bronchospasm, inability to detect hypoglycemia, fatigue, bradycardia
Direct vasodilators (hydralazine, minoxidil)	Used in difficult-to-control hypertension	Headaches, fluid retention, tachycardia
CCBs (dihydropyridines: amlodipine, nifedipine, isradipine)	Drugs of first choice for posttransplant hypertension; antagonize afferent arteriolar vasoconstriction	Nondihydropyridines increase cyclosporine and tacrolimus levels. Edema, tachycardia, and headache
ACE inhibitors (captopril, enalapril, lisinopril, quinapril)	Useful in CHF, postmyocardial infarction, native kidney hypertension	May increase creatinine and K^+ and decrease hematocrit. Cough, hyperkalemia
ARBs (losartan, candesartan, irbesartan)	Similar to ACE	Similar to ACE

Table 1. Antihypertensive class of drug, advantages in kidney transplant recipients, and side effects. ACE: angiotensin-converting enzyme; ARB: angiotensin receptor blocker; CCB: calcium channel blocker; CHF: congestive heart failure; IHD: ischemic heart disease.

hyperlipidemia is characterized by increased total cholesterol, increased or normal high-density lipoprotein (HDL), and increased low-density lipoprotein (LDL) with or without hypertriglyceridemia [60].

Of the available immunosuppressive agents, sirolimus causes the greatest increase in serum lipids [61]. CsA and corticosteroids also increase lipid values, whereas MMF and tacrolimus have a limited effect on posttransplant lipids. While prednisone increases total cholesterol, it also increases HDL. Corticosteroid withdrawal protocols demonstrate an improvement in total cholesterol; this is offset by a reduction in HDL. In one study, total cholesterol decreased by 17%, and HDL cholesterol fell by 18% [62].

The treatment of hyperlipidemia to decrease cardiovascular risk is well established in the general population. Although there are no long-term, prospective, controlled studies in the transplant literature, it is reasonable to infer that transplant recipients will also benefit from cholesterol-lowering agents. In the 1980s, treatment of hyperlipidemia was tempered by reports of rhabdomyolysis in heart transplant recipients treated with gemfibrozil and lovastatin while on CsA immunosuppression [63].

Rhabdomyolysis and myopathy appear to be more frequent in transplant recipients who receive CsA or tacrolimus. The likely explanation is interference of hydroxymethylglutaryl-coenzyme A (HMG-CoA) reductase inhibitor metabolism of calcineurin inhibitors in the cytochrome P450 system in the liver. This may cause higher blood levels of the drugs (CsA or tacrolimus). Because of the higher incidence of musculoskeletal side effects in transplant recipients, most transplant physicians start with lower doses of CsA or tacrolimus in transplant recipients receiving these drugs.

The most appropriate first-line pharmacologic agents for the treatment of hyperlipidemia are HMG-CoA reductase inhibitors, since the most common lipid abnormality is elevated total cholesterol and LDL. Fibrates can be used, but close monitoring is required, especially when used in conjunction with HMG-CoA inhibitors. Bile acid sequestrants are effective, but are poorly tolerated by most patients. These agents may also interfere with immunosuppressive drug absorption. Nicotinic acid is an ideal drug to reduce triglycerides, increase HDL, and lower cholesterol, though its use may result in hyperuricemia and hyperglycemia. A list of the available classes of lipid-lowering drugs and special

Drug class	Lipid effects	Clinical considerations in transplant recipients
HMG-CoA reductase inhibitors	↓↓ LDL ↑ HDL ↓ Triglycerides	Metabolized in P450 system. Cyclosporine and tacrolimus can increase half-life, increasing the risk of myopathy or rhabdomyolysis
Bile acid sequestrants	↓↓ LDL ↑ HDL ↔ Triglycerides	May interfere with absorption of immunosuppressive drugs. Poorly tolerated by most patients
Nicotinic acid	↓ LDL ↑↑ HDL ↓↓ Triglycerides	May aggravate hyperuricemia induced by cyclosporine or tacrolimus. May cause or worsen hyperglycemia
Fibrates	↓ LDL ↓ Cholesterol ↑ HDL ↑↑ Triglycerides	Increased incidence of myopathy and rhabdomyolysis with concomitant use of HMG-CoA reductase inhibitors

Table 2. Classes of available lipid-lowering agents, effect on lipid values, and considerations in transplant recipients. CoA: coenzyme A; HDL: high-density lipoprotein; HMG-CoA: hydroxymethylglutaryl coenzyme A; LDL: low-density lipoprotein. ↓: decreased; ↑: increased; ↔: no change.

considerations for their use in transplant recipients is shown in **Table 2**.

Most transplant recipients fall into the highest cardiovascular risk categories described by the National Cholesterol Education Program III [64]. However, the goals for LDL (<100 mg/dL) and triglycerides (<150 mg/dL) may not be achievable in some transplant recipients because of intolerance to therapy, or unacceptable risk of myopathy or rhabdomyolysis.

Cardiovascular disease

The incidence of cardiac events in the renal failure population is at least 10 times higher than that in the general population. Cardiovascular disease is responsible for approximately 40% of all deaths following successful kidney transplantation [65]. This is unsurprising, since at least 50% of the transplant population has diabetes mellitus and pre-existing vascular disease. In an analysis of US Renal Data System data from 1987 to 1997, 42% of deaths occurred in patients with a functioning graft [66]. Reducing mortality from cardiovascular disease could improve long-term kidney allograft survival.

A recent study examined risk factors for IHD events >1 year after successful kidney transplantation [67]. Important risk factors for IHD events included diabetes, smoking, history of rejection, bilateral nephrectomy for polycystic kidney disease, low serum albumin, proteinuria, and hyperlipidemia. Many of these risk factors are potentially remediable, but there have been no long-term studies of risk-factor modification in kidney transplant recipients. Although there are no long-term studies of screening for cardiovascular disease in asymptomatic transplant recipients following transplantation, it seems prudent to screen those recipients with multiple risk factors.

Transplant recipients with known coronary artery disease prior to transplantation who have undergone coronary revascularization, percutaneous transluminal coronary angioplasty (PTCA), or stent placement exhibit similar survival rates to recipients without known pretransplant coronary artery disease [68]. Herzog et al. reported a 43% reduction in death or myocardial infarction in recipients with coronary artery bypass grafting compared with PTCA ($P < 0.001$) [68]. There was no appreciable difference in coronary artery events in recipients with PTCA or stenting.

Bone disease

Bone disease is a significant problem in the long-term kidney transplant recipient. The etiology of posttransplant bone disease is complex and multifactorial. Most transplant recipients have one or more risk factors for bone disease at the time of transplant, and many patients already have significant bone disease.

Diabetes, pretransplant use of corticosteroids, gonadal failure, diuretics, poor nutritional status, and immobility all contribute to pretransplant bone disease. It is estimated that 8%–49% of patients with kidney failure have osteoporosis at the time of transplantation [69]. Renal osteodystrophy from hypothyroidism, osteomalacia, a dynamic bone disease, or osteosclerosis also confer risk for bone loss prior to transplantation [69].

Bone loss is accelerated after transplantation. Two separate studies have reported a 7% loss of bone mineral density (BMD) in the lumbar spine at 6 months posttransplantation [70,71]. The bone loss is multifactorial, but glucocorticoid therapy, CsA, and tacrolimus have been implicated in its pathogenesis. Subclinical hyperparathyroidism and hypogonadism are also prevalent in the posttransplant setting.

Because most bone loss occurs in the immediate posttransplant period, BMD should be determined early in the posttransplant course. In patients with significant bone disease, measurements of parathyroid hormone, 25-hydroxyvitamin D, thyroid function, and serum testosterone (in men) should be performed. Therapy should include calcium (1500 mg/day), vitamin D (400–800 mg/day), and hormonal supplementation, if appropriate. Treatment with bisphosphonate (alendronate 70 mg/week or risedronate 30 mg/week) should also be instituted [72,73].

Posttransplant infection

Because of the need for life-long immunosuppression, transplant recipients are at risk for significant infectious complications. At least 80% of patients develop an infectious complication posttransplant. Most opportunistic infections occur relatively early in the posttransplant period, when immunosuppressive therapy is most aggressive. Most later infections are due to the same etiologies as in the general population. Urinary tract infection is the most common late infection, followed by upper respiratory tract infection.

In transplant recipients without an obvious source of infection, a diligent search for opportunistic and less common infections needs to be undertaken. Of the late opportunistic infections, cytomegalovirus (CMV) is the most common. Late CMV presents with fever and a falling total white blood count. The gastrointestinal tract is the most affected organ system when a patient presents with CMV infection.

The underlying kidney disease also predisposes transplant recipients to certain infections. Patients with diabetes mellitus often present with fever and infection from complications arising from foot ulcers, cellulitis, and osteomyelitis. Transplant recipients with polycystic kidney disease may present with abdominal pain and fever from diverticulitis. Recipients with a history of reflux or a neurogenic bladder frequently have recurrent urinary tract infections. It is important to remember that any significant infection may reactivate CMV.

Recipients with fever of unknown origin may have posttransplant lymphoproliferative disease (PTLD), which is described in detail in the following section.

Malignancy

Long-term transplant recipients have a 3- to 5-fold higher incidence of *de novo* malignancies than the general population [74]. Lymphoma and skin cancer are the most common malignancies detected in long-term transplant recipients. It is unclear whether solid tumors, such as lung, breast, colon, prostate, or cervical cancer, are more common in long-term transplant recipients than in the general population.

PTLD commonly presents with unexplained fever or asymptomatic lymphadenopathy. The risk of developing PTLD is 1%–3% [75]. The diagnosis is often associated with rising serum lactate dehydrogenase and elevated β_2-microglobulin. Biopsy of affected lymph nodes or involved tissues is required for a definitive diagnosis. Treatment involves reducing immunosuppression, antiviral therapy with ganciclovir (or acyclovir in Epstein–Barr virus-positive cases), and rituximab therapy. In nonresponders or patients with progressive disease, chemotherapy and radiotherapy may be necessary.

Skin cancer is the most common posttransplant malignancy. The risk of developing skin cancer increases by 4- to 7-fold in regions with limited sun exposure. In areas with significant sun exposure, there is 20-fold increase in risk compared with the local population [75]. Most skin cancers are basal cell carcinomas, and are easily treated with local excision. Rarely, Kaposi's sarcoma occurs in the posttransplant recipient. Papilloma virus may be a causative agent in some transplant recipients with skin cancer.

Risk factors for the development of *de novo* cancers in kidney transplant recipients have been analyzed in a single-center study [76]. Risk factors for the development of cancer were:

- age ≥60 years relative risk [RR] 3.81, $P < 0.001$ compared with age <45 years)
- age ≥45 and <60 years RR 2.0, $P = 0.007$ compared with age <45 years)
- pretransplant splenectomy (RR 1.87, $P < 0.016$)
- pretransplant invasive cancer (RR 2.38, $P = 0.015$)
- cigarette smoking (each 10 pack-years smoked at transplant, RR 1.12, $P = 0.016$)

Patients with type 1 diabetes mellitus had the lowest risk of developing cancer (RR 0.19, $P = 0.015$). Because of the higher incidence of cancer in the at-risk population, aggressive screening is recommended for early detection. Routine colonoscopy, mammography, and screening for cervical cancer are recommended.

Conclusion

Long-term survival (>10 years) was once the exception for kidney transplant patients. Over the past 2 decades, improvements in immunosuppression have led to increased patient and graft survivals, and it is common to see successful long-term transplant recipients. There are two major issues in the long-term management of transplant patients. The first is prolongation of allograft function for as long as possible. Transplantation is a life-prolonging procedure, and failure of the allograft results in a mortality of 60% at 5 years in patients who return to dialysis [77]. Adequate attention to kidney function, compliance, and immunosuppressive drug levels, and prompt intervention when allograft dysfunction occurs, requires close observation in the posttransplant period.

The second major issue is preventing premature mortality, since kidney graft survival depends on patient survival. A total of 42% of deaths occur with a functioning graft, and most are due to cardiovascular disease. Effective prevention includes optimal blood pressure control and aggressive treatment of lipid abnormalities. The other major preventable cause of death in transplant patients is malignancy. Routine screening for colon, breast, and skin cancer is recommended.

References

1. Cecka JM. The UNOS Scientific Renal Transplant Registry – 2000. In: Cecka JM, Terasaki PI, editors. *Clinical Transplants 2000*. Los Angeles: UCLA Immunogenetics Center, 2001:1–18.
2. United States Renal Data System. *USRDS 2002 Annual Data Report: Atlas of End-Stage Renal Disease in the United States*. Bethesda, MD: National Institutes of Health, National Institute of Diabetes and Digestive and Kidney Diseases, 2002.
3. United States Renal Data System. Excerpts from the USRDS 2001 Annual Data Report: Atlas of End-Stage Renal Disease in the United States. *Am J Kidney Dis* 2001; 38(Suppl. 3):S53–S68.
4. United States Renal Data System. Excerpts from the USRDS 2001 Annual Data Report: Atlas of End-Stage Renal Disease in the United States. *Am J Kidney Dis* 2001; 38(Suppl. 3):S117–S134.
5. Cicciarelli J, Iwaki Y, Mendez R. The influence of donor age on kidney graft survival in the 1990s. In: Cecka JM, Terasaki PI, editors. *Clinical Transplants 1999*. Los Angeles: UCLA Immunogenetics Center, 2000:335–40.

6. LaRosa JC, He J, Vupputuri S. Effect of statins on risk of coronary disease: a meta-analysis of randomized controlled trials. *JAMA* 1999;282:2340–6.
7. Ross SD, Allen IE, Connelly JE et al. Clinical outcomes in statin treatment trials: a meta-analysis. *Arch Intern Med* 1999;159:1793–802.
8. Lewis SJ, Moye LA, Sacks FM et al. Effect of pravastatin on cardiovascular events in older patients with myocardial infarction and cholesterol levels in the average range. Results of the Cholesterol and Recurrent Events (CARE) Trial. *Ann Intern Med* 1998; 129:681–9.
9. Caro J, Klittich W, McGuire A et al. The West of Scotland coronary prevention study: economic benefit analysis of primary prevention with pravastatin. *BMJ* 1997;315:1577–82.
10. Hebert PR, Gaziano JM, Chan KS et al. Cholesterol lowering with statin drugs, risk of stroke, and total mortality. An overview of randomized trials. *JAMA* 1997;278:313–21.
11. Saag KG, Emkey R, Schnitzer TJ et al. Alendronate for the prevention and treatment of glucocorticoid-induced osteoporosis. Glucocorticoid-Induced Osteoporosis Intervention Study Group. *N Engl J Med* 1998;339:292–9.
12. Homik J, Cranney A, Shea B et al. Bisphosphonates for steroid induced osteoporosis. *Cochrane Database Syst Rev* 2000;(2):CD001347.
13. Boutsen Y, Jamart J, Esselinckx W et al. Primary prevention of glucocorticoid-induced osteoporosis with intravenous pamidronate and calcium: a prospective controlled 1-year study comparing a single infusion, an infusion given once every 3 months, and calcium alone. *J Bone Miner Res* 2001;16:104–12.
14. Kasiske BL, Chakkera HA, Louis TA et al. A meta-analysis of immunosuppression withdrawal trials in renal transplantation. *J Am Soc Nephrol* 2000;11:1910–7.
15. Ahsan N, Hricik D, Matas A et al. Prednisone withdrawal in kidney transplant recipients on cyclosporine and mycophenolate mofetil—a prospective randomized study. Steroid Withdrawal Study Group. *Transplantation* 1999;68:1865–74.
16. Matas AJ, Ramcharan T, Paraskevas S et al. Rapid discontinuation of steroids in living donor kidney transplantation: a pilot study. *Am J Transplant* 2001;1:278–83.
17. Racusen LC, Solez K, Colvin RB et al. The Banff 97 working classification of renal allograft pathology. *Kidney Int* 1999;55:713–23.
18. Racusen LC, Solez K, Colvin R. Fibrosis and atrophy in the renal allograft: interim report and new directions. *Am J Transplant* 2002;2:203–6.
19. Fellstrom B. Nonimmune risk factors for chronic renal allograft disfunction. *Transplantation* 2001;71(11 Suppl.):SS10–SS16.
20. Massy ZA, Guijarro C, Wiederkehr MR et al. Chronic renal allograft rejection: immunologic and nonimmunologic risk factors. *Kidney Int* 1996;49:518–24.
21. Paul LC. Chronic allograft nephropathy: an update. *Kidney Int* 1999;56:783–93.
22. Hariharan S. Long-term kidney transplant survival. *Am J Kidney Dis* 2001;38 (Suppl. 6):S44–S50.
23. Weir MR, Ward MT, Blahut SA et al. Long-term impact of discontinued or reduced calcineurin inhibitor in patients with chronic allograft nephropathy. *Kidney Int* 2001; 59:1567–73.
24. McGrath JS, Shehata M. Chronic allograft nephropathy: prospective randomised trial of cyclosporin withdrawal and mycophenolate mofetil or tacrolimus substitution. *Transplant Proc* 2001;33:2193–5.
25. Weir MR. Methods and outcomes of calcineurin inhibitor reduction or withdrawal in patients with chronic allograft nephropathy after the first year posttransplantation. *Transplant Proc* 2001;33(4 Suppl.):19S–28S.
26. Hausberg M, Kosch M, Hohage H et al. Antihypertensive treatment in renal transplant patients—is there a role for ACE inhibitors? *Ann Transplant* 2001;6:31–7.

27. Ersoy A, Dilek K, Usta M et al. Angiotensin-II receptor antagonist losartan reduces microalbuminuria in hypertensive renal transplant recipients. *Clin Transplant* 2002; 16:202–5.
28. Lin J, Valeri AM, Markowitz GS et al. Angiotensin converting enzyme inhibition in chronic allograft nephropathy. *Transplantation* 2002;73:783–8.
29. Schnuelle P, van der Heide JH, Tegzess A et al. Open randomized trial comparing early withdrawal of either cyclosporine or mycophenolate mofetil in stable renal transplant recipients initially treated with a triple drug regimen. *J Am Soc Nephrol* 2002;13:536–43.
30. Weir MR, Anderson L, Fink JC et al. A novel approach to the treatment of chronic allograft nephropathy. *Transplantation* 1997;64:1706–10.
31. Gonzalez Molina M, Seron D, Garcia del Moral R et al. Treatment of chronic allograft nephropathy with mycophenolate mofetil after kidney transplantation: a Spanish multicenter study. *Transplant Proc* 2002;34:335–7.
32. Myers BD, Ross J, Newton L et al. Cyclosporine-associated chronic nephropathy. *N Engl J Med* 1984;311:699–705.
33. Olyaei AJ, de Mattos AM, Bennett WM. Nephrotoxicity of immunosuppressive drugs: new insight and preventive strategies. *Curr Opin Crit Care* 2001;7:384–9.
34. Bloom IT, Bentley FR, Garrison RN. Acute cyclosporine-induced renal vasoconstriction is mediated by endothelin-1. *Surgery* 1993;114:480–7.
35. Marsen TA, Weber F, Egink G et al. Differential transcriptional regulation of endothelin-1 by immunosuppressants FK506 and cyclosporin A. *Fundam Clin Pharmacol* 2000;14:401–8.
36. Bobadilla NA, Tapia E, Jimenez F et al. Dexamethasone increases eNOS gene expression and prevents renal vasoconstriction induced by cyclosporin. *Am J Physiol* 1999;277:F464–F471.
37. Bobadilla NA, Gamba G, Tapia E et al. Role of NO in cyclosporin nephrotoxicity: effects of chronic NO inhibition and NO synthases gene expression. *Am J Physiol* 1998;274:F791–F798.
38. Shihab FS, Yi H, Bennett WM et al. Effect of nitric oxide modulation on TGF-β1 and matrix proteins in chronic cyclosporine nephrotoxicity. *Kidney Int* 2000;58:1174–85.
39. Vieira JM Jr, Noronha IL, Malheiros DM et al. Cyclosporine-induced interstitial fibrosis and arteriolar TGF-β expression with preserved renal blood flow. *Transplantation* 1999;68:1746–53.
40. Johnson RW, Kreis H, Oberbauer R et al. Sirolimus allows early cyclosporine withdrawal in renal transplantation resulting in improved renal function and lower blood pressure. *Transplantation* 2001;72:777–86.
41. Anjum S, Andany MA, McClean JC et al. Defining the risk of elective cyclosporine withdrawal in stable kidney transplant recipients. *Am J Transplant* 2002;2:179–85.
42. Heim-Duthoy KL, Chitwood KK, Tortorice KL et al. Elective cyclosporine withdrawal 1 year after renal transplantation. *Am J Kidney Dis* 1994;24:846–53.
43. Smith SR, Minda SA, Samsa GP et al. Late withdrawal of cyclosporine in stable renal transplant recipients. *Am J Kidney Dis* 1995;26:487–94.
44. Smak Gregoor PJ, de Sevaux RG, Ligtenberg G et al. Withdrawal of cyclosporine or prednisone six months after kidney transplantation in patients on triple drug therapy: a randomized, prospective, multicenter study. *J Am Soc Nephrol* 2002; 13:1365–73.
45. MacPhee IA, Bradley JA, Briggs JD et al. Long-term outcome of a prospective randomized trial of conversion from cyclosporine to azathioprine treatment one year after renal transplantation. *Transplantation* 1998;66:1186–92.
46. Burke JF Jr, Pirsch JD, Ramos EL et al. Long-term efficacy and safety of cyclosporine in renal-transplant recipients. *N Engl J Med* 1994;331:358–63.

47. Cosio FG, Pelletier RP, Falkenhain ME et al. Impact of acute rejection and early allograft function on renal allograft survival. *Transplantation* 1997;63:1611–5.
48. Humar A, Kerr S, Gillingham KJ et al. Features of acute rejection that increase risk for chronic rejection. *Transplantation* 1999;68:1200–3.
49. Vincenti F, Jensik SC, Filo RS et al. A long-term comparison of tacrolimus (FK506) and cyclosporine in kidney transplantation: evidence for improved allograft survival at five years. *Transplantation* 2002;73:775–82.
50. Opelz G, Wujciak T, Ritz E. Association of chronic kidney graft failure with recipient blood pressure. Collaborative Transplant Study. *Kidney Int* 1998;53:217–22.
51. Laskow DA, Curtis JJ. Post-transplant hypertension. *Am J Hypertens* 1990;3:721–5.
52. Curtis JJ. Hypertension following kidney transplantation. *Am J Kidney Dis* 1994;23:471–5.
53. Schwenger V, Zeier M, Ritz E. Hypertension after renal transplantation. *Ann Transplant* 2001;6:25–30.
54. Guidi E, Menghetti D, Milani S et al. Hypertension may be transplanted with the kidney in humans: a long-term historical prospective follow-up of recipients grafted with kidneys coming from donors with or without hypertension in their families. *J Am Soc Nephrol* 1996;7:1131–8.
55. Huber A, Heuck A, Scheidler J et al. Contrast-enhanced MR angiography in patients after kidney transplantation. *Eur Radiol* 2001;11:2488–95.
56. van den Dorpel MA, Zietse R, Ijzermans JN et al. Prophylactic isradipine treatment after kidney transplantation: a prospective double-blind placebo-controlled randomized trial. *Transpl Int* 1994;7(Suppl. 1):S270–S274.
57. Midtvedt K, Hartmann A, Foss A et al. Sustained improvement of renal graft function for two years in hypertensive renal transplant recipients treated with nifedipine as compared to lisinopril. *Transplantation* 2001;72:1787–92.
58. Venkat Raman G, Feehally J, Coates RA et al. Renal effects of amlodipine in normotensive renal transplant recipients. *Nephrol Dial Transplant* 1999;14:384–8.
59. Kobashigawa JA, Kasiske BL. Hyperlipidemia in solid organ transplantation. *Transplantation* 1997;63:331–8.
60. Pirsch JD, D'Alessandro AM, Sollinger HW et al. Hyperlipidemia and transplantation: etiologic factors and therapy. *J Am Soc Nephrol* 1992;2(12 Suppl.):S238–S242.
61. Morrisett JD, Abdel-Fattah G, Hoogeveen R et al. Effect of sirolimus on plasma lipids, lipoprotein levels, and fatty acid metabolism in renal transplant patients. *J Lipid Res* 2002;43:1170–80.
62. Hricik DE, Schulak JA. Metabolic effects of steroid withdrawal in adult renal transplant recipients. *Kidney Int Suppl* 1993;43:S26–S29.
63. East C, Alivizatos PA, Grundy SM et al. Rhabdomyolysis in patients receiving lovastatin after cardiac transplantation. *N Engl J Med* 1988;318:47–8.
64. Expert Panel on Detection, Evaluation, and Treatment of High Blood Cholesterol in Adults. Executive summary of the third report of the National Cholesterol Education Program (NCEP) Expert Panel on Detection, Evaluation, and Treatment of High Blood Cholesterol in Adults (Adult Treatment Panel III). *JAMA* 2001;285:2486–97.
65. Kasiske BL. Cardiovascular disease after renal transplantation. *Semin Nephrol* 2000; 20:176–87.
66. Ojo AO, Hanson JA, Wolfe RA et al. Long-term survival in renal transplant recipients with graft function. *Kidney Int* 2000;57:307–13.
67. Kasiske BL, Chakkera HA, Roel J. Explained and unexplained ischemic heart disease risk after renal transplantation. *J Am Soc Nephrol* 2000;11:1735–43.
68. Herzog CA, Ma JZ, Collins AJ. Comparative survival of dialysis patients in the United States after coronary angioplasty, coronary artery stenting, and coronary artery bypass surgery and impact of diabetes. *Circulation* 2002;106:2207–11.
69. Shane E, Epstein S. Transplantation osteoporosis. *Transplant Rev* 2001;15:11–32.

70. Casez JP, Lippuner K, Horber FF et al. Changes in bone mineral density over 18 months following kidney transplantation: the respective roles of prednisone and parathyroid hormone. *Nephrol Dial Transplant* 2002;17:1318–26.
71. Julian BA, Laskow DA, Dubovsky J et al. Rapid loss of vertebral mineral density after renal transplantation. *N Engl J Med* 1991;325:544–50.
72. Giannini S, Dangel A, Carraro G et al. Alendronate prevents further bone loss in renal transplant recipients. *J Bone Miner Res* 2001;16:2111–7.
73. Arlen DJ, Lambert K, Ioannidis G et al. Treatment of established bone loss after renal transplantation with etidronate. *Transplantation* 2001;71:669–73.
74. Zeier M, Hartschuh W, Wiesel M et al. Malignancy after renal transplantation. *Am J Kidney Dis* 2002;39:E5.
75. Penn I. Cancers in renal transplant recipients. *Adv Ren Replace Ther* 2000;7:147–56.
76. Danpanich E, Kasiske BL. Risk factors for cancer in renal transplant recipients. *Transplantation* 1999;68:1859–64.
77. Kaplan B, Meier-Kriesche HU. Death after graft loss: an important late study endpoint in kidney transplantation. *Am J Transplant* 2002;2:970–4.

Abbreviations

ACE	angiotensin-converting enzyme
APC	antigen-presenting cell
ARB	angiotensin receptor blocker
AST	American Society of Transplantation
ATG	antithymocyte globulin
AUC	area under the curve
BMD	bone mineral density
BMI	body mass index
CAN	chronic allograft nephropathy
CCB	calcium channel blocker
CD40L	CD40 ligand
CMV	cytomegalovirus
CNS	central nervous system
CoA	coenzyme A
CsA	cyclosporin A
CT	computed tomography
CTL	cytotoxic T lymphocyte
CTLA	common T-leukocyte antigen
DGF	delayed graft function
DTH	delayed-type hypersensitivity
EBV	Epstein–Barr virus
ESRD	end-stage renal disease
FasL	Fas ligand
GFR	glomerular filtration rate
HAART	highly active antiretroviral therapy
HBeAg	hepatitis B envelope antigen
HBsAb	hepatitis B surface antibody
HBsAg	hepatitis B surface antigen
HCV	hepatitis C virus

HDL	high-density lipoprotein
HHV	human herpes virus
HIV	human immunodeficiency virus
HLA	human leukocyte antigen
HMG	hydroxymethylglutaryl
HSV	herpes simplex virus
HTLV	human T-lymphotropic virus
IFN	interferon
Ig	immunoglobulin
IHD	ischemic heart disease
IL	interleukin
LDL	low-density lipoprotein
MGU	monoclonal gammopathy of undetermined significance
MHC	major histocompatibility complex
MMF	mycophenolate mofetil
MRA	magnetic resonance angiography
mTOR	mammalian target of rapamycin
NFAT	nuclear factor of activated T cells
NK	natural killer
Pap	Papanicolaou
PKD	polycystic kidney disease
PTCA	percutaneous transluminal coronary angioplasty
PTLD	posttransplant lymphoproliferative disease
PVD	peripheral vascular disease
RANTES	regulated on activation, normal T-cell expressed and secreted
RAS	renal artery stenosis
RR	relative risk
SMA	superior mesenteric artery
TB	tuberculosis
TCR	T-cell receptor
TGF	transforming growth factor
TOR	target of rapamycin
UNOS	United Network for Organ Sharing
USRDS	United States Renal Data System
VZV	Varicella–Zoster virus

Index

A

ABO blood typing 70
acne 50
acute rejection 5–8, 99
  clinical correlates 31–4
  effector mechanisms 29–31, **30**
  resolution 31
  withdrawal of steroids 47
acyclovir 61, 110
adrenergic inhibitors, side-effects 104
age at transplantation 68–9
alendronate 108
alloantibodies 15, 17–18
  posttransplant responses 33–4
allograft nephropathy *see* chronic allograft nephropathy (CAN)
allografts
  age at transplantation 68–9
  defined 14
  injury and salvage 93
  long-term, management 98–9
  outcomes 4–8
  revascularization **85**, **87**, **88**
  see also acute rejection; chronic rejection
allorecognition, T cells 18–20, 33
allosensitization 67
alopecia 50
anemia 50
aneurysm, mycotic 91, 93

angiotensin-converting enzyme (ACE) inhibitors 100
  vs. CCBs 103
  side-effects 103, **104**
angiotensin receptor blockers (ARBs) 100
  side-effects **104**
antibodies
  acute rejection, effector mechanisms 29
  alloantibodies 15, 17–18, 33–4
  anti-CD25 antibodies 40–3
  anti-CD40L antibodies 25
  antilymphocyte antibodies 8
  antimurine (OKT3) 41–2
  induction therapy 40–3
  monoclonal antibodies 40–2
  polyclonal antibodies 42–3
  structure 17–18
antigen-presenting cells (APCs) **15**, 16, **21**
  costimulation 24–6
antihypertensive agents, summary **104**
antimetabolites 47–9
antimurine antibodies, OKT3 42
antithymocyte globulin 42–3
antiviral agents 61, 110
aorto-iliac disease, evaluation 63
arterial stenosis, complication of transplantation 92–3, 102–3
arterial thrombosis 92–3
atenolol, side-effects **104**
ATG (antithymocyte globulin) 42–3
azathioprine 48
  side-effects **50**

B

B cells 14, 27–8
  activation 27–8
  alloantibodies 15, 17–18
  memory, resolution, acute rejection 31
basiliximab 41, 43

beta-adrenergic blocking agents
posttransplant hypertension 103
side-effects **104**
bile acid sequestrants, hyperlipidemia 105, **106**
biopsy, living-related donors 72
bisphosphonate 108
bone disease 107–8

C

C4d 32
cadaver donors 4
graft half-lives **5**
organ preservation 82
procurement
heart-beating 81–2
nonheart-beating 82
selection criteria 80–2
calcineurin inhibitors
chronic therapy 44–6, 100–2
conversion strategy (avoidance/contraindications) 9, 98, 100
and HMG-CoA reductase inhibitors 105
offsetting by CCBs 103
side-effects **50**
see also cyclosporine; tacrolimus
calcium channel blockers (CCBs) 103, **104**
vs. ACE inhibitors 103
calyceal blowout 91
cancer 50
cancer-free waiting times **58**
contraindications to transplantation 57
posttransplant risk factors 109–10
screening 65–6
candesartan, side-effects 104
captopril *see* angiotensin converting-enzyme (ACE) inhibitors
cardiovascular disease
CAD/IHD investigation 62, 107
mortality in graft recipients 7–8, 106–7

CD3-binding OKT3 41–2
CD4 and CD8 molecules 18–19, **21**, 22
CD28 ligand 24
CD40 ligand 24, 27
  anti-CD40L antibody 25
cellular immune responses 14, 18–34
chemokines 28–9
cholesterol *see* hyperlipidemia
chronic allograft nephropathy (CAN) 6–8, 39–40, 99–100
  at 1 year 99
  conversion to rapamycin therapy 51
  mechanisms **33**
  rejection, clinical correlates 31–4
  treatment 100
chronic rejection *see* chronic allograft nephropathy
clonidine **104**
complications of surgery 90–3
  infections 91, 95
  long-term 97–110
  transplant nephrectomy 95
  urologic complications 91–2
  vascular complications 92–3
coronary artery disease (CAD/IHD)
  investigations 62, 107
  risk factors 107
corticosteroids
  action 47
  avoidance/contraindications 9, 98
  and hyperlipidemia 105
  side-effects 47, **50**
CTLA-Ig 24
cyclosporine (CsA)
  chronic therapy 100–1
    rhabdomyolysis 105, **106**
    vs. tacrolimus 102
  side-effects 45, **50**
  toxicity 100–1

see also calcineurin inhibitors
cytomegalovirus infection 109
contraindications to transplantation 61

D

daclizumab 41
diabetes mellitus 50
and bone disease 108
cancer, posttransplant risk factors 109–10
dialysis vs. transplantation, numbers 2
infections 109
diuretics, side-effects **104**
doxazocin **104**
dual transplantation 86–7

E

end-stage renal disease (ESRD), and peripheral vascular disease 62–3
Epstein–Barr virus infection, posttransplant 110
ethics, living-related donors 75

F

fibrates, hyperlipidemia 105, **106**
fibrosis, nonimmune factors 34
FK-506 (tacrolimus) 46
see also tacrolimus
FK-binding proteins 49
FTY720 28

G

ganciclovir 61, 110
gastrointestinal symptoms 50
gemfibrozil, rhabdomyolysis 105
genitourinary dysfunction, evaluation 63
gingival hyperplasia 50
graft rejection *see* allograft; acute rejection; chronic rejection
Gregoir–Lich ureteroneocystostomy 86

H

hematoma formation 50, 90–2
hematuria, following nephrectomy 95
hemolytic–uremic syndrome (HUS) 50
hepatitis B/C, contraindications to transplantation 60
hirsutism 50
HIV infection, contraindications to transplantation 56–9
human leukocyte antigen (HLA) molecules 3, 15, **17**
  alloantibodies 15, 17–18
humoral immune responses 14, 17–22, 27–8
humoral immunity 17–18
hydralazine **104**
hyperlipidemia 50, 103–5
  corticosteroids 105
  treatment 105, **106**
hypertension 50
  living-related donors 71
  posttransplant 102–3
    beta-blockers 103
    CCBs 103

I

immune response stages 14–34
  activation
    B cells 27–8
    T cells 24–7
  allorecognition 16–24
  effector functions 29–31
  migration of T cells 28–9
immunology 13–34
  graft rejection mechanisms 29–31
  transplantation immunity **15**
immunophilins 44
immunosuppression/immunosuppressive drugs 8–11, 39–51
  future trends 9–10
  immunologic tolerance 10–11
  induction therapy 8, 40–3

maintenance therapy 43–51
see also specific drugs
Imuran (azathioprine) 47–8, **50**
induction therapy 40–3
antilymphocyte antibodies 8
monoclonal antibodies 40–2
polyclonal antibodies 42–3
infections
complication of transplant nephrectomy 95
complication of transplantation 91, 108–9
contraindications to transplantation 56–63
inflammation 33
insomnia 50
interferons, production by T cells 27, 28
interleukins
drug inhibition 44
IL-2, CD25 T-cell receptor 40–1
IL-2 receptor pathway 26–7
irbesartan, side-effects 104
isografts 14

L

labetalol, side-effects **104**
lactate dehydrogenase (LDH) 109–110
lamivudine 60
Ledbetter ureteroneocystostomy 86
leukopenia 43, 50
lipid-lowering drugs 105, **106**
lisinopril
vs. nifedipine 103
see also angiotensin converting-enzyme (ACE) inhibitors
liver, combined transplantation 89
living-related donors 2–3
absolute contraindications 73–4
ethics 75
expanded evaluation 70–3
list of tests **71**

graft half-lives **5**
limited initial evaluation 69
selection criteria 83
surgical procurement
laparoscopic nephrectomy 84
open nephrectomy 83–4
long-term complications of surgery 97–111
losartan, side-effects 104
lovastatin, rhabdomyolysis 105
lymphocele 90–1
lymphoproliferative disease, posttransplant 109–10

M

maintenance therapy 43–51
major histocompatibility complex (MHC) 14, 16, **17**
malignancy 50
posttransplant 109–10
see also cancer
mammalian target of rapamycin (mTOR) 49
marginal (cadaver) donors 4
metalloproteinases 29
metoprolol, side-effects **104**
minor transplantation antigens 22–4
minoxidil **104**
monoclonal antibodies 40–2
mortality in graft recipients
and allograft life expectancies 2, 97–8, **99**
cardiovascular disease 7–8, 106–7
mycophenolate mofetil (MMF) 47–9, 100
side-effects 49, **50**
see also immunosuppressive drugs
mycotic aneurysm 91, 93
myopathy, CsA chronic therapy 105, **106**

N

Neoral (cyclosporine) 45
nephrectomy

laparoscopic 84
open 83–4
of transplant 93–5
nephropathy, chronic allograft 6–8
neurological symptoms 50
nicotinic acid, hyperlipidemia 105, **106**
nifedipine
vs. lisinopril 103
see also calcium channel blockers (CCBs)
noncompliance 67

O

obesity 50
and transplant prognosis 66
organ preservation 82
Orthoclone Muromonab-CD3 (OKT3) 41–2
osteoporosis 50, 108

P

pancreas, combined transplantation 89
pediatric transplantation 89–90
en bloc 87–8
peripheral vascular disease, investigation in ESRD 62–83
peritonitis, catheter removal pretransplantation 59–60
polyclonal antibodies 42–3
polycystic kidney disease, living-related donor with 72
posttransplant lymphoproliferative disease (PTLD) 109–110
prednisone *see* corticosteroids
pre-emptive transplantation 67–8
Prograf (tacrolimus) 46
see also tacrolimus
pulmonary function tests, living-related donors 72

R

RANTES molecule 28–9
rapamycin *see* sirolimus
recipient evaluation 55–68

contraindications to transplantation **56**, 56–64
recommendations to recipients 66–7
rescreening 65–6
routine vs. elective investigations **64**
summary 64–5
renal artery
bypass 93
extension with saphenous vein 85–6
stenosis and pseudostenosis, complication of transplantation 92–3, 102–3
retransplantation 88–9
revascularization **85**, **87**, **88**
rhabdomyolysis
CsA chronic therapy 105, **106**
gemfibrozil 105
lovastatin 105
risedronate 108
rituximab 110

S

Sandimmune *see* cyclosporine
saphenous vein, extension of renal artery 85–6
Simulect (basiliximab) 41
sirolimus 49–51, 100
anticancer properties 51
hyperlipidemia 104
side-effects **50**
substance abuse 67
surgery 79–96
cadaver donor procurement
heart-beating 80–2
nonheart-beating 82
complications 90–3
living-related donor procurement
laparoscopic nephrectomy 84
open nephrectomy 83–4
transplant nephrectomy 93–5

see also transplantation

T

T cells
activation 24–7
costimulation 24–6
IL-2 receptor pathway 26–7
allorecognition of MHC–peptide complexes 18–20
apoptosis 10, 29
CD4 and CD8 molecules 18–19, **21**, 22
chronic rejection 32
differentiation 27
effector mechanisms, acute rejection 29–31
immune responses 14–34
indirect recognition of MHC–peptide complexes 20–2
memory, resolution, acute rejection 31
migration 28–9
T-cell receptors (TCRs) 18–20
TCR–MHC–peptide complex 20
tacrolimus 46, 101
vs. cyclosporine (CsA) 102
side-effects **50**
see also calcineurin inhibitors
target of rapamycin (TOR) 49
terazosin **104**
thrombocytopenia 43, 50
thrombotic thrombocytopenic purpura 50
Thymoglobulin (antithymocyte globulin) 42–3
transplant nephrectomy
absolute/relative indications 93–4
complications 94–5
transplantation
life expectancies 97–8, **99**
dialysis vs. transplantation 2
living donor vs. cadaver 97–9
with other organs 89
pediatric 89–90

en bloc 87–8
pre-emptive 68
retransplantation 88–9
single kidney 85–6
two (dual) 86–7
transplantation immunity, mechanisms **15**
tuberculosis, contraindications to transplantation 59

U

ureteral implantation 86
ureteral stenting 91–2
ureteroneocystostomy, anterior/posterior 86
urologic complications 91–2

V

vascular complications 92–3
vascular-vesical fistla 94
vasculopathy/fibrosis, nonimmune factors 34
vasoconstriction, cyclosporine-related 45
vasodilators, side-effects **104**
venous thrombosis, complication of transplantation 92–3

Z

Zenapax (daclizumab) 41